PENGUIN BOOKS

Stand By Me

Sir John Kirwan, one of the most devastating wingers that world rugby has ever seen, was an All Black from 1984 to 1994, playing 63 tests. Following his playing career, JK went on to coach the Italian and Japanese national rugby teams, and is now the Head Coach of the Auckland-based Super Rugby franchise the Blues.

JK has also become an advocate for depression awareness in New Zealand, fronting a high-profile TV campaign and authoring the bestselling memoir *All Blacks Don't Cry* in 2010. In 2012, he was appointed a Knight Companion of the New Zealand Order of Merit, for services to mental health and rugby.

JK is a dedicated husband and father of three teenagers.

JOHN KIRWAN

Stand By Me

Helping your teen through tough times

with Elliot Bell and Kirsty Louden-Bell
and Margie Thomson

PENGUIN BOOKS

Stand By Me provides suggestions to assist adults to identify and respond to indications of anxiety and depression (and related concerns) in adolescents. These suggestions should never preclude seeking assistance from health professionals. A general practitioner is often the best first port of call – they can help determine whether the young person has mental health concerns and, if so, what treatment or follow-up options are available or appropriate. The GP may offer treatment themselves, and/or may suggest referral to one or more of the following: a public mental health service; a non-governmental organisation (NGO); a psychiatrist, clinical psychologist, or other therapist in private practice; or a guided self-help resource.

The specific treatments endorsed in *Stand By Me* are based on current evidence. As new research is produced, an evidence base for additional treatments may emerge. Some of the individual cases referred to in *Stand By Me* are informed by the actual clinical work of the authors. Others, where quotations are included, are drawn from interviews undertaken for *Stand By Me* with teens, parents and siblings whose lives have been affected by mental illness. While the quotes are direct, specific details and identifying information have been modified to protect the privacy of these individuals.

About the co-authors

Dr Elliot Bell is a registered clinical psychologist. He trained at Victoria University of Wellington, and has worked clinically in private practice and in local District Health Board mental health services. He currently works as a lecturer and researcher at the University of Otago's School of Medicine and Health Sciences in Wellington, and has a private practice in central Wellington where he sees clients. Elliot is active in the New Zealand College of Clinical Psychologists, currently serving as Vice President. His professional interests include cognitive behavioural treatments of depression, anxiety and schizophrenia; positive psychology; and measurement in psychology.

Kirsty Louden-Bell is also a registered clinical psychologist, and graduated from Victoria University of Wellington in 1995. She has worked in a range of mental health settings in the public sector, as well as in private practice, and has experience in training and presenting, both nationally and internationally. She has a passion for youth and youth work, and since 2001 has been involved through Clinical Advisory Services Aotearoa (CASA) as both a clinician and the manager of a nationwide programme aimed at identifying and managing risk in young people at risk of suicide.

Elliot and Kirsty live in Wellington and have two sons and a daughter.

***

Margie Thomson has had a long career working in magazines and newspapers, including as a feature writer and books editor for the *New Zealand Herald*, and feature writer and book reviewer for *Your Weekend*. She has co-written many books, including John Kirwan's *All Blacks Don't Cry*, Ray Columbus's *The Modfather*, Malcolm Rands's *Ecoman*, three titles with Kelvin Cruickshank, and – with Angela McCarthy – *The Hungry Heart: Anorexia and Bulimia*. She has a Master's in Creative Writing and won the inaugural James Wallace Publication Prize in 2013.

Margie is married to James and has three children. She lives in Auckland.

PENGUIN BOOKS
Published by the Penguin Group
Penguin Group (NZ), 67 Apollo Drive, Rosedale, Auckland 0632,
New Zealand (a division of Penguin New Zealand Pty Ltd)
Penguin Group (USA) Inc., 375 Hudson Street,
New York, New York 10014, USA
Penguin Group (Canada), 90 Eglinton Avenue East, Suite 700, Toronto,
Ontario, M4P 2Y3, Canada (a division of Penguin Canada Books Inc.)
Penguin Books Ltd, 80 Strand, London, WC2R 0RL, England
Penguin Ireland, 25 St Stephen's Green, Dublin 2,
Ireland (a division of Penguin Books Ltd)
Penguin Group (Australia), 707 Collins Street, Melbourne,
Victoria 3008, Australia (a division of Penguin Australia Pty Ltd)
Penguin Books India Pvt Ltd, 11, Community Centre,
Panchsheel Park, New Delhi – 110 017, India
Penguin Books (South Africa) (Pty) Ltd, Block D, Rosebank Office Park,
181 Jan Smuts Avenue, Parktown North, Gauteng 2193, South Africa
Penguin (Beijing) Ltd, 7F, Tower B, Jiaming Center, 27 East Third Ring Road
North, Chaoyang District, Beijing 100020, China

Penguin Books Ltd, Registered Offices: 80 Strand,
London, WC2R 0RL, England

First published by Penguin Group (NZ), 2014
1 3 5 7 9 10 8 6 4 2

Designed and typeset by Shaun Jury
Photography by Alistair Guthrie
Printed and bound in Australia by Griffin Press, an Accredited
ISO AS/NZS 14001 Environmental Management Systems Printer

ISBN 978-0-143-57063-9

A catalogue record for this book is available from the
National Library of New Zealand.

www.penguin.co.nz

MIX
Paper from
responsible sources
FSC www.fsc.org FSC® C009448

Contents

Prologue

I'm a dad and I'm scared.

I've got three great kids who are all teenagers now. I say to my youngest son, 'How was school today?' 'Good,' he says.

I say to my other son, after 45 minutes with the careers counsellor: 'How was it, mate?'

'Good!'

'So what are you going to do for a job?'

'Too many questions, Dad.'

My 19-year-old daughter calls from Italy where she's a professional volleyballer. She's in tears because she's lonely and wants to come and live with us in New Zealand. We end the Skype call and all I can do is worry.

I had a mental illness, but I still don't know how to parent for mental wellness. I want to parent so that if things are going wrong for my kids I'll see it and know what to do.

I'm a solutions guy. I'm a rugby coach. If someone isn't playing well I can look at their game and go: his scrummaging or high-ball skills need work. When I was a butcher's apprentice I knew how to give the customer what they wanted. If I was a maths teacher I could tell if you didn't understand why x plus y equals z, and I would know what to do to help. But when it comes to guarding the mental health of our children, what are the answers? How do I know what's going on in their heads, in their lives? How do I talk to them?

As part of my research for this book I spoke to a range of young people and their parents or caregivers, asking questions and seeking everyday, real insights.

Sophie: For people our age things are constantly changing. Your relationship with your parents changes. At school your subjects change, your teachers change, your friends are changing – and if you fall out with your friend group, you're really in trouble.
Ellen: Your social scene, getting exposed to drugs and things in your social life . . .
Jim: Most people bottle it up and keep it in until it eventually overflows.

JK: The story I've told about my own mental illness was that it hit me like a truck when I was 23. Out of the blue I had a panic attack. I told no one. I couldn't explain it – my life looked so good; I had nothing to complain about. I was lucky! I had no right to be sad: I was an All Black, at the top of my game, I'd played really well in the World Cup . . . And in fact sometimes when I played, in that pre-depression period, I felt something like euphoria – it was like a massive high before the storm. Yet inside of me I had doubts about how good I was. I was always supercritical of myself. That was part of what made me a good player, but I understand now that it was also out of control, and underneath it all I had a massive fear of failure. I wasn't good enough. *I'm overrated. It's all a lie.* Over the next three years the panic increased and I developed full-on depression, until eventually came the terrible, terrifying day when I couldn't get out of bed.

Fear is often the monkey in the room, messing everything up. Inside myself I had all this fear but I didn't deal with it, and so I had what people might call a mental breakdown.

Depression took my confidence and, as a rugby player, I don't believe I ever really got my confidence back 100 percent.

It seemed to come from nowhere, but now I realise there were early warning signs – things that went right back to my childhood. For instance, I got homesick in Hunua – yeah, I know, it sounds like a sad country song, and it was. I was 10 or 11, with all my mates, out in this beautiful place with nothing to do but have fun for a few days – but I was sobbing. I wanted to go home, and Mum had to drive out and get me. Mum said, 'You're just homesick.' I reckon a lot of people thought I was a real sook. But was it the first signs of anxiety? Is that the kind of thing that we as parents should be aware of? If it is, how do we parent it? Counsel it? Do whatever we need to do?

As parents, we're the first doctor – you know, like in those Vicks ads – yet I don't think we ever have the confidence to say: *I did everything I could*.

In our culture, which is a pretty hard culture, a lot of people would probably say to a homesick kid, or as a rugby mate said to me when I was falling apart in Italy: 'Just harden up.' But I don't think that's the attitude if we want to create resilience in our young people. I said it in my book *All Blacks Don't Cry*, and I'll say it again: maybe it's time we tried the opposite – 'Just soften up.'

At that camp in Hunua they would have had a first-aid box filled with sticking plasters and bandages and disinfectant. But what about the first-aid box for a child who's crying from a fear of the unknown, and feeling helpless and afraid? What would that look like?

Resilience. That's the buzzword of the moment – but what does it mean and how can we achieve it in our kids so that they're able to roll through all the ups and downs of life?

I've got so many questions, and I'm not an expert. I often say, I'm just a butcher making shit up. I want what you want: a good relationship with my children; to not be afraid that I'm missing something important in their lives that's causing them problems; to help them in the right way. Dad always said you don't know until they're about 26 what kind of job you've done with your parenting. I want my kids, when they reach that age, to think they had great parents, and that I didn't let them down.

For 10 years now I've been involved in campaigns to raise awareness about depression. People tell us that these campaigns are helping a lot. Doctors say people are less afraid to come and see them and tell them how they're feeling, and get some help. Awesome. But what freaks me out is that mental health among our young people is still not good. We have one of the highest youth suicide rates in the world. There's something we're not doing right. And you know what?

Every conversation I have about this subject – with health professionals, with parents – leads down a pathway not just to relatively simple matters like parenting techniques, but to really big subjects like the kind of society we've created, the kind of values we have. It comes back to the uncertainty that we as parents and caregivers have about our role with our kids. How much do we have the right to ask about? When should we step up, and when should we step back? We need courage and confidence; and we need to think about our values.

British children's author Philip Pullman says: 'After nourishment, shelter and companionship, stories are the thing we need most in the world.' I believe that by sharing our stories we can learn from each other. A lot of people – kids, parents and caregivers – have generously shared their stories for this book. No one's story is exactly the same, but you'll be surprised at how many similarities there are. We all live in the same world, after all. I can't tell you how many times, since publishing *All Blacks Don't Cry*, people have said to me, 'It was like reading about myself.' Hundreds, maybe thousands of times I've been told that.

Reaching out and sharing my story is one of the best things I ever did, as it's put me in touch with so many amazing people – people who have been in a very dark place, as I was, but who have found their way back to the land of the living. You'll see from many of the stories in this book that, without exception, people who have had mental illness feel that they have emerged stronger than they were before. And this is one of the complex mysteries of life: that, with the right kind of support, hard times shape us – 'refine us', as one of our dads puts it – and make us who we are.

I'm not making light of it. There are far too many people – and far, far too many kids – who don't make it back to the land of the living.

Having anxiety and depression was the worst thing that ever happened to me, and at the time I didn't see how things could ever get better. But I made it through and I'm glad to be the person I am now – definitely with more self-knowledge and more compassion for others.

Clinical psychologists Dr Elliot Bell and Kirsty Louden-Bell, my collaborators in this book, tell us that one way to make ourselves feel better is to be grateful and to do things for other people – this is part of what is called 'positive psychology'. Wow. That's really radical advice because it goes against the way society pushes us – to want *more* all the time, and to be so busy we don't have time to look outside our own little lives. Elliot and Kirsty's point is interesting because it suggests a contradiction between social pressure and what it takes to be well. In the 'I' society that we live in, people say, 'I won't do something for someone else; I'll do it for me.' But I saw a great comment online recently: 'When the "I" is replaced by "we", even illness becomes wellness.'

For mental wellness, you probably need to behave a bit differently from how society is telling you to behave. Society is saying *go fast*, and mental health is saying *slow down*. Slow the treadmill down.

For kids, these issues are especially pertinent. What's it like to be a kid today? We explore that throughout this book, and I can tell you, it's not like it was when I was a boy. There's lots more pressure on kids to know at a very young age what they want to study, what they want to become – 'the bigness of it all,' as one 13-year-old put it to me recently. Everything's competitive. There's social media, which constructs a kind of false world where it looks like everyone else's life is happy and perfect and popular. Teenagers are surrounded by drugs and alcohol and encouraged to grow up and make their own decisions when they're scarcely out of primary school.

We've given them this world. How can we help them through it?

Today I went and sat in the sun with a cup of coffee. I don't do that often enough. I tried to be still, to feel the sun on my face, to really taste the coffee. I've learned that these simple things keep me well. *Slow down.*

I realise I've been rushing. I rush to work in the morning; it's 35 minutes from home to work, and I feel like I'm pushing the whole way. I'm not even late but I'm rushing. Why? It's a state of mind. *Shit, I'm busy.* Well, hang on a minute. Why don't I just relax and enjoy it? I know I could seriously get depressed again unless I make a conscious effort to say to myself, *hang on*. And that makes me realise: it's not just *what* I'm doing, it's *how* I'm living while I do it. There are two approaches to driving to work in the morning, and neither gets me there any sooner. There are lots of things I can't change, but it is within my power to change the way I drive to work in the morning.

Being present in the moment is part of what psychologists call mindfulness. It's an increasingly recognised technique that contributes to wellbeing. There are programmes trialling teaching this to kids in primary school. Brilliant – it should be part of the curriculum.

When researching *Stand By Me*, as well as looking at stories of how people got unwell, we asked them, 'What did you do to get well? What do you do to stay well, to thrive?'

I'm drawing on a whiteboard. I draw a house like a child might draw one – a box with a triangle on top. Hey, I'm not an artist! Inside this house there are rooms. I see the house; my son sees only the room that he's in at the moment. He mistakes the room he's in for the whole house.

Remember what it was like? We were all there once. For adolescents, their whole life is in that moment, and it's only as they get older that they can bring in that bigger picture. They don't yet have the knowledge or the experience that helps them cope. And that's where we parents come in, listening and talking and not fobbing them off with 'she'll be right' or 'plenty of other fish in the sea'. Age brings perspective.

It's not that long ago that my own dad gave me some advice on this. I was grown up, but trying to decide whether to take the contract to coach the Japanese rugby team. He said: 'When you're my age and look back on life, three years is nothing.' He was seeing the whole house. Even then, he was encouraging me to walk through my own house and check out some of those other rooms.

One of the things that's happened to me since I began campaigning for mental health is that I sometimes speak with the mums and dads of children who are suffering, or with the young person themselves. Mostly I just share my own story, let them know they're not alone. Or I connect them with an appropriate mental health professional, let them know it's OK to get help and to talk.

That's the freaky thing about mental illness – in a single moment they can't see tomorrow, and tomorrow is the whole house. Today is just the room they're stuck in.

Mental illness brings so much pain and disappointment. Often, these brave young people who have been through depression miss out on a lot of the normal things along the way. Education, for instance: for some kids, their struggle with depression means they leave school without their qualifications. But at the age of 19 or 20 they can't go, 'I'm uneducated.' They need to acknowledge, 'I'm well. I can tackle the world again.'

People have done it – I know people who have gone back to school at 60! It's not over. It's never over.

But this comes back to society and the linear push-through. Growing up is not about straight lines. When depression comes along, you sometimes have to drop your hopes and dreams and just love the child you've got. Layla says this really well about her 13-year-old daughter Christie: 'When a child has mental illness, a lot of things that they and you hoped for might no longer be possible. Some of your dreams for your child must die or be put on hold – certainly, they must change . . . But you strip that away, and the child you have is the real child.' That's the child you need to stand by and love.

And that's why we've called this book *Stand By Me*. Love is a powerful theme. As parents, it's our main theme.

I've always said that marriage is conditional – that is, I expect something back from Fiorella, and she expects things from me. We're two people who have come together, we're in love, but there are expectations.

Parenting, though, is different: it's unconditional. I have unconditional love for my kids and just want the best for them.

But love is a verb, not just a feeling. With Elliot and Kirsty's help we'll try and get to the bottom of what love looks like when it's confronted by one of the biggest challenges of all: a child desperately ill with anxiety or depression, who simply doesn't seem like the child who was there before.

Mental illness isn't just something that happens to individuals. When one family member is sick, the whole family rocks on its foundations. Getting well is a family matter. Psychiatrist Peter McGeorge, former New Zealand Mental Health Commissioner, acknowledged this when he said: 'Everyone knows that families are important. However understanding their importance in the recovery of family members who have experienced mental illness is only relatively recent.'

Equipping parents with the knowledge and courage to be active and supportive in their children's lives, especially when anxiety and depression come to call, is an important goal of this book – and a recurring theme in many of the stories told here.

When I say I'm a dad and I'm scared, I really mean: I'm a dad and I'm looking for answers. I'm looking for answers from the professionals and I'm looking for answers from the other kind of expert: the kids, mums, dads and other caregivers who have been there, holding each other's hands to hell and back.

Stand by me. Let's take the journey together.

Introduction

> The man who moves a mountain begins by carrying away small stones.—Confucius

Stand By Me has grown out of the concerns I have as a parent, and which I believe I share with most other parents and caregivers. I wanted a resource that would tell me how to talk to my children about anxiety and depression; help me as a parent to know how to recognise possible early signs of depression or anxiety; and give me skills to talk to my children about what's going on in their lives and to offer suggestions on how to look after their mental health.

My friends Dr Elliot Bell and Kirsty Louden-Bell, who are both clinical psychologists as well as being the parents of three children, are my go-to people for the latest professional thinking about mental illness and mental health in adolescents. This book is an equal partnership between them and me. Elliot works at the University of Otago, was an adviser for *All Blacks Don't Cry*, and also worked with me on the depression.org website. Kirsty has worked in both adult and child mental health, and is the clinical manager of a programme for young people at risk of suicide.

I see this book as a conversation of many voices – kids, parents, caregivers, youth workers, health professionals – all sharing their experiences and insights. We've spoken to kids who have suffered depression or anxiety, and who have generously given us their time to reflect on their experiences and treatment and how they have been shaped by their illness. We've spoken to parents and caregivers about the challenges of helping their young person through tough times.

We've written this book for people like us – parents and other adults who are concerned about anxiety or depression in their own or others' teenage children. We think, though, that if any adolescent picks it up there will be plenty that will resonate with them, too.

We were also conscious that, apart from illnesses such as depression and anxiety, life throws up challenges for every young person – the changing dynamic between them and their parents, friendships, love, freedom, fitting in, alcohol and drugs, and so on – and that young people deal with these challenges in myriad ways, often positive, sometimes not. With this in mind, I went and spoke with a couple of classrooms of awesome kids in Years 12 and 13 at Mt Albert Grammar – a big multicultural Auckland secondary school – and their words are scattered throughout the book.

Stand By Me is not a how-to parenting manual – there are lots of great parenting books out there by New Zealand and international experts (we list some of these authors in the Resources section at the back of the book). Nor is it a step-by-step treatment manual – again, we suggest some books and websites of that type for specific mental health problems in our Resources section. It's kind of in the middle – raising the questions, journeying together alongside the professionals, those experienced at working with young people, and those parents and young people with lived experience, to figure out what some of the answers might be, and how we can stand by each other.

It's also important to note that this is not a clinical book, and it in no way replaces clinical advice. It is meant as a guide to how to recognise when you might need such advice, and a resource for parents who are wondering what they can do – typically alongside professional help.

This is how we're going to move through this book. We'll start by getting a sense of what's going on for adolescents today, both in society and inside their own heads – inside that famous object, the teenage brain. Then we're going to get to know anxiety and depression – what they are, what they look like, as well as some of the scary things that can be associated with them, such as eating disorders, self-harm, drugs and alcohol misuse, and suicide. We'll look at treatments and therapies. And finally we'll look at recovery and prevention – how by encouraging wellness and resilience in our kids we can help them avoid risky patterns of thought and behaviour that can lead to anxiety and depression.

Lastly, Elliot and Kirsty have put together some useful lists of further material you can turn to – books and online resources that offer more specialised and detailed information, as well as online support groups and online treatment programmes.

There's a lot of exciting initiatives going on in the area of mental health awareness and support. This book hopes to be a small part of that bigger picture, or an entry point for people like me who might not know where to start.

The concept of recovery has transformed the field of mental health. Most people with mental illness get better if they can get help. But there is also hope for people who have long-term difficulties. It is increasingly recognised that recovery is about living well in the presence or absence of mental illness.

Acknowledgements – JK, Elliot and Kirsty

Ehara taku toa i te toa takitahi, engari he toa takitini. This powerful whakatauki (Maori proverb) sums it up well: 'My strength is not mine alone, it is the strength of many.'

This book – like our wellness – exists because of the strength of many. From the outset, we want to stress how grateful we are to the courageous, inspiring individuals and families who said yes to being part of this book. These people opened their hearts and shared their powerful stories with us. Their names and identities are confidential, but they know who they are!

Of course we must also acknowledge our own families, friends, colleagues, and communities – those who stand by us and are part of our strength.

Others who have contributed to this book also warrant special mention. We would like to thank consultant psychiatrist Dr Lyndy Matthews for sharing her invaluable knowledge on the use of psychiatric medications, and for contributing her broader wisdom on working with and talking to families about mental illness. We would also like to express our great appreciation to clinical psychologist Denise Steers for her support, and for bringing her expertise in child and adolescent psychology to early reviews of the manuscript. Our special thanks are also extended to Jeremy Sherlock, commissioning editor at Penguin, for shepherding this project to its completion with constant enthusiasm and patience; and to Leanne McGregor at Penguin for her very thorough and always helpful input. Finally, and most of all, we wish to express our particular gratitude to Margie Thomson, freelance writer extraordinaire. Margie, you not only did much of the heavy lifting in the writing and interviews for the book, but you always ensured that the tone was real and the voices authentic. We cannot thank you enough.

To you, the readers who have picked up this book, we hope that the questioning, conversations and stories of courage within will give you strength and encouragement on your journey.

Note: The main reports that we reference throughout this book are: *Youth'12 Overview: The Health and Wellbeing of New Zealand Secondary School Students in 2012* (referred to as the Youth'12 Report) – part of an ongoing research project into our secondary school students that's done every five years or so; *Improving the Transition: Reducing Social and Psychological Morbidity During Adolescence* (referred to as the Gluckman Report) from the Prime Minister's Chief Science Adviser, Professor Sir Peter Gluckman; *Te Rau Hinengaro: The New Zealand Mental Health Survey* (referred to as the New Zealand Mental Health Survey); and two important longitudinal studies – the Dunedin Multidisciplinary Health and Development Study, and the Christchurch Health and Development Study (referred to respectively as the Christchurch and Dunedin longitudinal studies) – each of which are tracking more than 1000 New Zealanders from birth and through their lives.

PART ONE

The Adolescent World

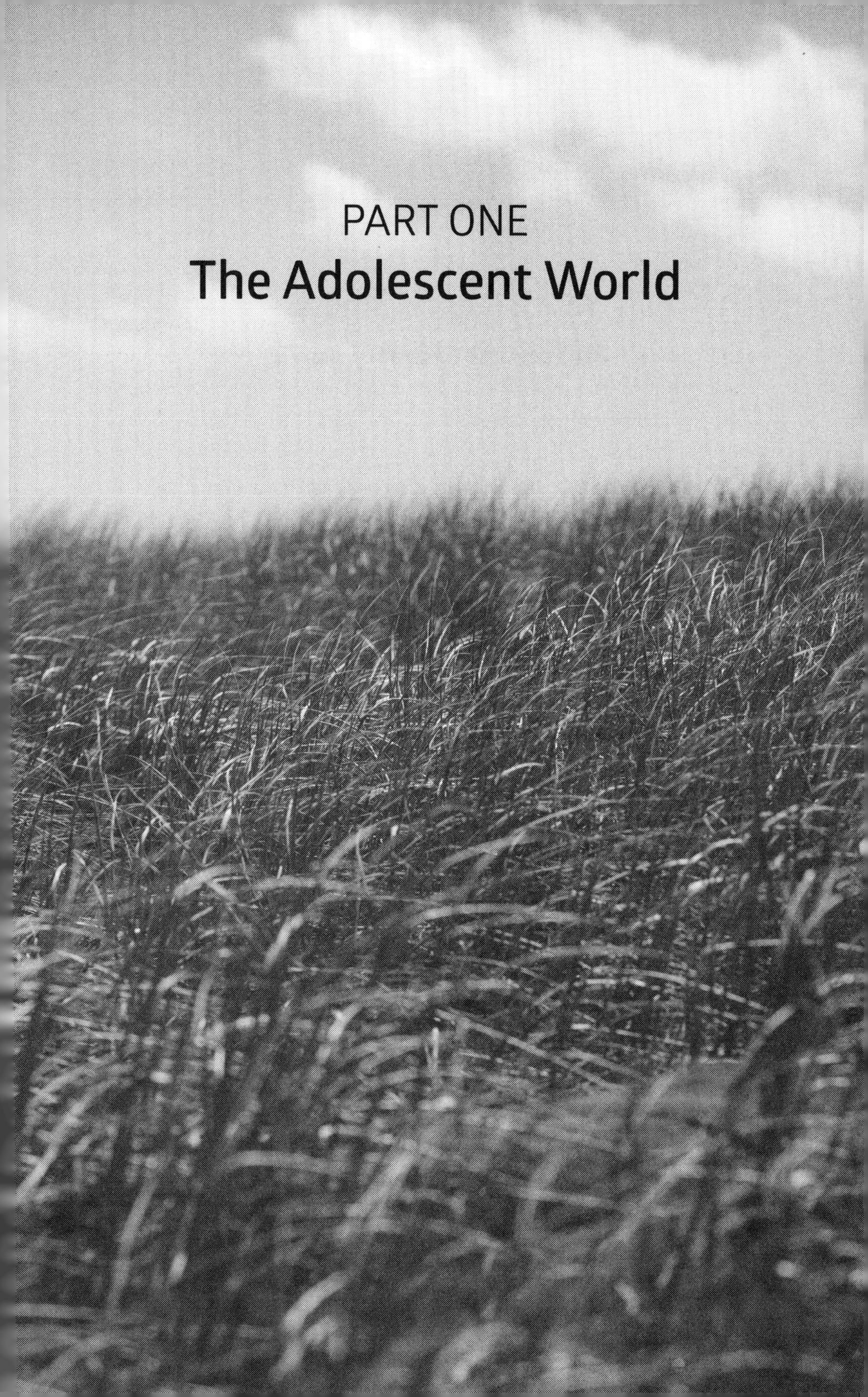

1.
Youth mental illness – adrift in stormy seas

> The New Zealand paradox: that is, New Zealand is a temperate, peaceful, ethical and developed nation in which children should flourish, yet it is actually one in which they experience some of the highest rates of adolescent morbidity and mortality in the OECD.—Gluckman Report, p. 54

JK: I asked some of the kids I spoke to if they felt that people understood their stress.

Flora: Your friends understand it.
Sophie: Your parents pretend they do.

JK: It's estimated that about one in five New Zealand kids will suffer from a depressive disorder by the time they're eighteen.

Mental illness has no prejudice – it can happen to anyone, rich or poor, black or white, male or female. But sadly, it's most common in young people between the ages of 15 and 24; and the number of young people affected rises steeply between the ages of 15 and 18 years. Depression is a leading risk factor for suicide, and New Zealand has one of the highest rates of teen suicide among OECD countries.

Most kids are resilient to the complexities of their social world and navigate their way through their teenage years without significant problems, and it's important to remember that. Nevertheless, when we look at the prevalence of mental illness among our teenagers, I think we all feel horrified. I know I do. I'm scared when I think of kids – not just my own, but any kids – going through what I went through with my mental illness.

Every classroom in the country will have at least someone who's struggling. Some of those struggling teens – like Jacob and Sean, whose stories we tell in this book – don't get help as early as they might have: bright young guys who nevertheless left school without any qualifications, thanks to the way depression played out in their young lives. And, of course, for every child who suffers, a family struggles as well.

We didn't use to think that kids could feel anxiety or depression. We used to think these were adult illnesses. How wrong we were. And there's plenty of evidence now to show that three-quarters of adults who suffer from anxiety or depression can trace their illness back into either their childhood or their adolescence. Like me. I didn't have my first panic attack until I was 23, but now I look back at myself as a child and I wonder: if I could have dealt with my anxiety then, could I have avoided the meltdown that was to come?

This is a huge wake-up call for our mental health services. Until recently, most public strategies to lower the rate of depression focused on adults. But we now know there is more to be gained by intervening earlier in people's lives. Thankfully, some new strategies are focused on youth – such as the Prime Minister's Youth Mental Health Project.

Personally, I'd like to see mental health on the curriculum in more schools. By teaching kids positive strategies we could prevent a lot of mental illness; and by building awareness – by simply talking more openly about it – we could combat the stigma and make it more likely that kids and their families would seek help, rather than battling on without treatment.

Jessica: I think people don't know much about depression. I had no idea it was so prevalent in New Zealand.

JK: If I was to say to you guys, we're going to screw up the national health curriculum and you're going to rewrite it, what would you write?

Scarlet: New Zealand-based, I think. We are involuntarily ignorant about big issues going on around us.
Moana: And I think it should be compulsory.
Adam: I'd make it more New Zealand-focused – issues that are big here, like mental health, obesity, alcohol.

Elliot: At the moment, according to the Gluckman Report, more than 80 percent of adolescent depression and anxiety disorders are left untreated. That's a recipe for future misery, because recurrence rates for depression are high – there's a 70 percent chance of a further episode within five years. Each depressive episode increases the probability of a further episode.

And that's a tragedy, because the good news is that *mental illness is treatable*. There are very effective treatments with very good rates of success, and there is a lot of support out there.

Also, the earlier it's identified and treatment can begin, the better the chance of success, and the better the chance that our young people will not experience further episodes.

Altogether, the studies indicate that anxiety and depression are increasing among our young people. It's not clear whether this is an actual increase, or whether it's a result of better screening and reporting. It may be a mixture of both. One thing we do know is: it's all around us. We've got work to do.

- One in five New Zealand kids will suffer from a depressive disorder by the time they're eighteen.
- The earlier it's treated the better.
- It can happen to anyone.
- Mental illness is treatable.

2.
Adding up the world

JK: I'm pretty insecure as a parent. I'm always saying to my wife, 'Are we doing the right thing?' We want our kids to get through to adulthood and for them to tell us we gave them the best shot – that we gave them our understanding. But that understanding is something we have to work at, because things are different now. Change is the order of the day. It boils down to this: kids are under more pressure at an earlier age than when I was a kid. There are important implications of this for parents.

> Given the dramatic technological changes that have taken place, it is almost impossible for the older generation to understand the context in which young people now live. It is an absolute mistake for an older generation to project their experiences onto this generation – the corollary being that a better understanding of young people in the 21st century is likely to be an important prerequisite for effective smoothing of the transition.—Gluckman Report, p. 6

I know that's how it's always been – the old 'generation gap' – but it seems more than ever that kids today are negotiating a fast and constantly changing world. The Gluckman and Youth'12 reports give us some insights into this:

- Cash is more readily accessible than to previous generations. Also, they are a key market segment, heavily targeted by media and advertisers.
- Alcohol is far more available than it was for previous

generations. Almost a quarter of high-school students are likely to binge drink in any given month. Teenage drinking is behind many of the other negative risk-taking behaviours that are far too common in New Zealand, such as unprotected and unwanted sex, drink-driving – and suicide.

- Bullying is a daily fact in our schoolyards. Six percent of school kids report being bullied at least once a week, and 9 percent are afraid someone will hurt or bother them. Twelve percent have received nasty or threatening messages on their phones, and 9 percent on internet sites. Later, two incredible young women, Nakita and Hayley, share with us their experiences of being bullied. I don't know about you, but what strikes me most about their stories, once I'd got over the cruelty, is their attitude of forgiveness and understanding. 'Hurt people hurt,' Nakita's mum says. These girls have wisdom beyond their years, and I hope people like them will be running the country one day.
- Some families are really struggling economically. The Youth'12 Report showed that 12 percent of young people say that their family often or always worries about not having enough money for food. It's harder to find part-time employment, and harder to get access to a family doctor. All these factors make it very challenging for families to be in a good state of physical and mental health; and studies show clearly that there is a greater risk of negative outcomes for adolescents from disadvantaged environments.
- Celebrity culture and social media are all around us, creating a fantasy world for kids to compare themselves to, and surrounding them with highly sexualised images that add loads of peer pressure and eat into their self-esteem. Exposure to celebrity culture is particularly problematic for teens, as those are the years in which young people are most actively trying to find their own identity. In fact, the main developmental task of adolescence relates to establishing identity. They're looking for role models. Celebrities are by definition successful, usually beautiful and wealthy – and

more than ever, they're right in front of our kids, onscreen, all the time. They look like they've got it all together. But they are impossible role models – never mind what we know about how many of these 'celebrities' are themselves breaking up inside.

- Thirty-three percent of high-school students have been hit or harmed by someone in the past year; 14 percent by an adult in their own home.
- Twenty percent of girls and 9 percent of boys in the past year have been touched in a sexual way or made to do unwanted sexual things; 57 percent didn't tell anyone about it.
- Four percent of high-school students aren't sure of their sexual identity; and 1 percent are transgender.
- Almost 30 percent divide their time between two or more homes.
- There is increasing ethnic diversity in our community, especially in the 12–24 age group. A growing number of high-school students say they belong to more than one ethnic group. While this brings great richness to our society, it carries its own challenges and conflicts for young people who are growing up as part of multiple worlds but who don't necessarily feel they belong in any.
- Really interesting to me is that while around 70 percent of young people questioned in the Youth'12 Report are happy with how they get along with their family, around 40 percent feel they don't get enough time with at least one of their parents. As parents we sometimes think our kids are more ready to do without us than they really are. They want us around, and they need us around – even though they don't always show it.

3.
The teenage brain – what's going on in there?

Jacob (now 20): I had really bad panic attacks at 13, and while I learned to deal with them, I was getting into a very unoptimistic state of mind that was the beginning of my depression. I got the drug habit early in my fourteenth year, which was interlinked with my social life, and to keep both I needed to give up some other stuff, which was family and my conscience. Being the druggie, rebellious kid was what I chose to be, and that was portrayed in the music I listened to, and what I wore, because that's how people could identify me as being that guy at school.

JK: Wow, we forget what it was like, don't we? *Who am I?* All those highs and lows. Figuring out who we wanted to be, being super-sensitive about how we looked, and whether or not we fitted in with our peers – who suddenly seemed so much more important than our parents.

Now, as parents ourselves, we're on the other side of the fence. Our kids grunt at us. They won't take off their headphones; they listen to music that's like an angry rant. Parents wonder, *what the hell is going on? Are they OK? Are they unwell? Are they suicidal? Or are they just normal?*

Elliot: The good news is, a lot of the irritating, even worrying adolescent behaviour that challenges our patience and drives us into self-doubt is absolutely normal.

Think about all the things adolescents are dealing with. They have to adjust to their sexually maturing bodies and all the feelings that go along with that; they often develop very intense feelings around relationships with friends, as well as the new territory of girlfriends and boyfriends; they are, crucially, figuring out their identity as individuals – and that means separating from their childhood identity which was so much dependent on their relationship with their parents. This means they have to renegotiate their relationships with their parents or caregivers. They have to find a way of expressing all this, and that's not easy because it's such complex, complicated territory.

Most of these milestones occur gradually over several years, in leaps and bounds or in stops and starts, and they are all part of the underlying developmental forces propelling adolescents towards maturity. But human development is increasingly viewed as a lifelong process, so as our adolescent children are doing their growing up, we – as parents and caregivers – are also facing challenges of our own. We have to cope with our teens' changes; we have to learn when to let go and when to move in more closely. We are learning and developing, too.

Biologically, part of the reason adolescents are moody is because their brain is changing so rapidly, and different bits of it are maturing at different rates. In recent years, science has advanced to give us a greater understanding of how the brain works and develops over time. Brain-scanning procedures have allowed us to look at the structure of the brain and to see how it changes through the years. What is apparent now is that the adolescent brain is not fully developed: it is still physically maturing until we're in our early twenties.

One aspect of these physical changes is the development of connections between the different areas of the brain. In teenage brains these connections develop unevenly. As a consequence, the capacity for strong emotional responses and emotionally driven behaviour tends to develop before problem-solving, critical thinking, impulse control, judgment and reasoning abilities. This, alongside hormonal changes, can explain some of the impulsiveness and associated risky behaviour in teens.

Risk-taking is one of the well-known characteristics of adolescence, and it's important to note that it's not a bad thing. It just needs to be channelled in the right way. Risk-taking when it comes to getting drunk and driving a car is clearly not good. The uncontrolled impulse that's involved in suicide is the greatest tragedy of all. But risk-taking when it comes to giving your all on the rugby field, or taking a role in the school play, or climbing a mountain with your school tramping club – those things all take guts and determination and all bring fantastic rewards. And they're all really, really good for helping your brain to grow and make the right connections.

JK: When you don't have control it's not risk-taking, it's stupidity. So what is risk-taking? Drink-driving? No, that's stupidity. Going away to a university in a different city? That's risk-taking. Going on an overseas trip with all the issues around safety and terrorism? That's risk-taking with sensibility. Doing drugs? That's stupidity.

Risk is different. Going surfing at Te Arai Point is positive risk-taking. You're 18, there's big surf, you've got the skills – or possibly not – but can you swim? Yes. That's positive risk.

We can't wrap kids in cotton wool.

Elliot: I agree, but for too many kids, negative risk-taking and/or anxiety and depression can lead to long-term negative consequences. Anxiety and depression are important factors in many problems, including failure at school and substance abuse – as we'll see later in the stories of Jacob and Sean.

Adolescent brains are highly vulnerable to alcohol and other drugs, and this is why the statistics relating to teenage binge drinking are so worrying. It can impair the hippocampus, which affects memory and learning. So our concern about teens drinking alcohol and using drugs is not just a moralistic concern – it's because these things can cause long-term damage, and can expose the young person to other risks such as depression, unwanted sex and pregnancy, drink-driving and so on.

Kirsty: Adolescence is a vital time for identity development. It's a time of individuation and separation. Kids are figuring out who they are, where they fit, what they are capable of and where they belong. As part of this they'll be adjusting to all the internal changes like those Elliot mentioned – adjusting their relationships and adjusting to their changing place in the world. Because there's so much going on anyway, young people and their families may not recognise signs of anxiety or depression, or may accept the symptoms as part of the usual experience of adolescents.

It's normal for adolescents to push the boundaries and experiment with their identity and take reasonable risks. But sometimes, if a child is struggling with underlying mental illness, these things can get out of control and become destructive. The problem is that untreated anxiety and depression can seriously jeopardise a young person's ability to negotiate the normal tasks of adolescence. They can affect schooling, relationships with peers and with parents. They can also have an effect on a young person's identity development: a young person with mental illness might relate to an identity that reflects their confusion, unhappiness and alienation. This can be self-perpetuating.

Jacob is an example of this. He got into drugs at a young age; and drugs and depression created a perfect storm that ensured he became an outsider at school. He was expelled and left school without any qualifications. 'This is who I am,' he would say angrily to parents and counsellors.

Early recognition of depression and anxiety helps to minimise their impact on these important stages of adolescent development.

- Adolescence is a time of massive change, both physically and in terms of relationships and identity.
- Adolescents' brains are still growing, affecting their mood and judgment.
- Positive risk-taking is an important part of adolescence – we need to create environments where they can explore and experiment without harming themselves and others.
- Because there's so much going on anyway, signs of anxiety or depression in a young person can be missed.
- Identifying and managing mental illness early is important so that it doesn't disrupt normal adolescent development.

4.
Calling all parents and caregivers

JK: How do we parent so that our kids are mentally healthy? How do we parent once mental illness has entered the house? Parents and caregivers – we need to step up. We seem to have lost confidence and become uncertain about our role, uncertain about our ability to influence our children's behaviour.

> Even within families with few risk factors, there is growing concern that parents feel unable to establish limits around their children's behaviour, particularly as they enter adolescence and the pressure of peers and the opportunities for risky behaviour increase. There is clearly a need to provide parents and caregivers with the skills and the resources that will help them to set effective limits on behaviour.—Gluckman Report, p. 9

As a parent, I find this is a very powerful message; and in a way it's one that's filled with hope. Problem is solution. If we can name our problems – and be really honest about them – that knowledge will point the way to a solution. In this book you'll see some amazing examples of parents who have stepped up and become fully involved in order to help their kids through mental illness.

Of course, we hate the idea of being over-controlling of our kids. My friend, psychiatrist Dr Lyndy Matthews, who contributed to the depression.org website, puts it this way:

Lyndy Matthews (psychiatrist): The natural response to illness in a child is for people to move in closer. It doesn't mean trampling on your child's rights. It doesn't mean putting a steel cage around

them. It means caring for them. It doesn't mean telling them what to do. It doesn't mean ordering them about. It means working with them collaboratively, and it means being there. *It means being there.* You're close in because she's sick. She's not sick because you're close in.

JK: I believe in hope. That's always been my message, and it's the thing that got me through my own dark times. Hold on to hope. And – this is something that Kirsty often says – if you're in the midst of depression and you can't find that hope in yourself, let someone else hold it for you. That's the role of parents and caregivers when a child is struggling with anxiety or depression and can't see that they're ever going to feel happy again. It's our job as parents to hold that hope for the child. We'll walk along with them, and we won't give up.

We've got work to do in understanding more about teenage anxiety and depression, and figuring out how we can help our kids. That's been my mission, and with Elliot and Kirsty's help we've got some great information and links to resources, some important advice and some exciting new things to think about.

- Parenting through adolescence is a challenge that we need to think through, particularly with regard to carefully setting boundaries.
- When a child is struggling with depression or anxiety, the parents need to step up and be present and involved.
- Parents need to work collaboratively with their children, walk alongside them and help them to hold on to hope.

PART TWO

The Dark Duo: Anxiety and Depression

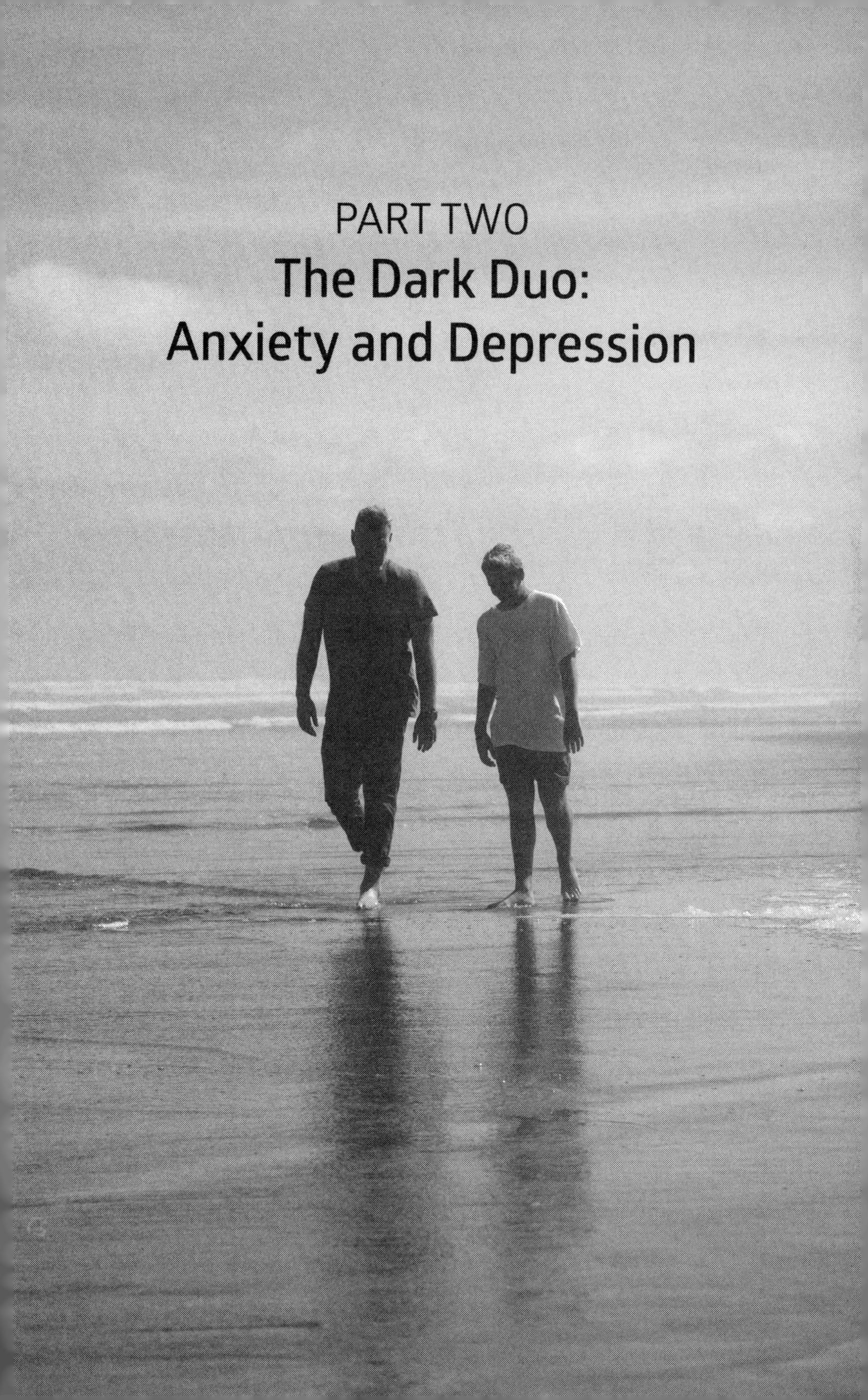

5.
What's wrong?

Kirsty: Tell me about depression.

Kate: Low self-esteem. It's a cycle.
Karl: One thing leads to another.
Flora: A black hole.

JK: Depression was a black monster that had come to live inside me. Every day I fought that black monster, and it exhausted me. I was in the grip of my darkest thoughts and feelings. The deep, messed-up thoughts – that I was going to do real harm to someone; that my life was a lie – had become completely real to me. Finally I ended up in bed, shaking and sweating and continually crying.

Depression is often described like that, isn't it? It's always 'dark'. Writers have described it as a 'thick, black paste', 'the muck of bleakness', 'the noonday demon', 'the black dog'. It is despair. It is 'relentless hopelessness'.

It's an illness, and I yell that from the hilltops. But what I've noticed is that people don't always believe it's an illness. They seem to think it's some sort of personality defect – as if someone feels this way because they've chosen to. Even I used to think that: I had the perfect life, so how dare I feel this way? I thought it was weakness. How can something that feels so emotional be an illness?

Elliot: Depression and anxiety *are* illnesses. Like physical conditions they have signs and symptoms, cause distress, and stop us functioning normally in our lives.

Depression is characterised by constant feelings of sadness or dullness or even – particularly in adolescents – anger and irritability. Thinking becomes pessimistic and negative.

Anxiety is characterised by overwhelming and irrational worry, dread and fear. Thinking becomes 'catastrophic' – focused on the worst-case scenario.

At their core, anxiety and depression are emotional states – types of fear and sadness – and as such are part of normal human experience. Fear helps keep us safe; anger motivates us to act; and sadness helps to show we care about things. But depressive and anxiety disorders are very different from everyday stress and the normal disappointments, sadness, fears and anxieties that come into all our lives from time to time.

We all know that adolescence is a time of acute emotion – it's part of this stage of human development and it's part of human life. But anxiety and depression are not just emotions. They are psychological states that we experience in our emotions, but also our thoughts, behaviours and physical reactions. They can get to the point where they are immensely disabling for the person experiencing them. They can be isolating and overwhelming for all of those involved.

Differentiating between the everyday human experience of anxiety and sadness, and depression and anxiety as mental health issues, can be a challenge for parents. In some ways it's a matter of degree. Beyond a certain point, anxiety and depression reduce our ability to function in daily life, and at that point they become mental disorders or illnesses. They both cause enormous mental distress.

The challenge is that, unlike with a physical illness such as a broken bone or diabetes, where a test can confirm the illness and then point to the best treatment, there is no physical test for depression or anxiety. There are, however, reliable diagnostic criteria that concentrate on the symptoms – what a person is actually experiencing – and the signs – what is observable in the person. And as JK noted, although people are very different in terms of what may be going on in their lives and contributing to their depression or anxiety, the symptoms are remarkably similar.

A qualified health professional such as a GP, psychiatrist or clinical psychologist is well equipped to give an accurate diagnosis and discuss treatment options. The important thing is that young people feel reassured about what is going on, and that there is help available for them.

Sean: Depression hit me when I was fifteen. I try and think about what triggered it and it stumps me. I think it has a lot to do with the fact that you're a teenager and you're thinking along the lines of, *is this what we're here for? Is this what life is? Is it going to be like this forever?*

I think a lot of it was to do with . . . on paper my life looked great, and that was something I really struggled with because on the inside I just felt something was there, building up.

You see so many people with terrible lives, a lot harder than I've had it, and I'm sitting here feeling bad about nothing. Nothing I could put my finger on. I felt guilty for feeling shit. I was also quite clouded, and my motivation was nonexistent. Lost, really, is a good way to put it.

Up until 13 I was really full of life. I was chirpy. But then I stopped doing most of the things I really enjoyed, even playing my drums. I didn't have the motivation or the energy. I'd go to play and be done in 10 seconds. I seemed to be in bed a lot. I dreaded school, and Mum was often having to ring and say I wasn't coming in.

Jacob: I spent a lot of time in my room, generally being quite lonely. You get used to being in your own company, thinking about yourself. Sometimes that's a good quality, but sometimes I think maybe I dug myself into a hole of depression through all my self-analysing.

Levi: A lot of the kids I see out on the street, deep down, they are depressed. They're just not going to show it because if you look weak or sad, people are going to come for you. So we hide it, we hide that depressed look, that depressed state. You go, *no, I'm fine, I'm a man, I can do it by myself.* That's how it is out there. If you look weak you will be weak, and someone will make you weak. They're not going to show you they're depressed. But deep down they are.

I was depressed because I didn't have a family to love, I didn't know who I was, I didn't have a sense of belonging. That's depressing stuff, but I had to show no weakness.

JK: My friend Brook Turner, a youth worker from ZEAL youth organisation (zeal.org.nz), makes a point to remind us that sometimes a young person might be struggling with normal sadness, and that's an opportunity for growth, not for medication.

Brook (youth worker): For some people a diagnosis will help. For others, I think we need to be careful. I knew one person who had a tragic loss. She was referred to a GP, who prescribed the antidepressant Prozac (fluoxetine). Yet there was a whole bunch of experiences that sat behind that feeling of depression, and in that moment that young person could very well just be in grief and not be depressed.

I would like us to give young people the language and the tools to be able to say, 'Actually, at this time I'm really struggling with feeling low. I don't feel I'm emotionally stable at the moment, but that doesn't necessarily mean I have a disorder.'

That's different from the kid who for 18 months has been struggling to get out of bed, who's got loving support around them, and where there's no obvious contributing factor to their emotional state of depression. That's a very different thing.

- Depression and anxiety are medical illnesses. They are different from everyday stress, disappointment and sadness.
- Despite people's individual differences, the symptoms of anxiety and depression are remarkably similar.
- Depression and anxiety reduce our ability to function in daily life.
- A health professional such as a GP, psychiatrist or clinical psychologist can give an accurate diagnosis and discuss treatment options.

6.
Depression and anxiety – distinct but related

JK: With me, my problems began with childhood anxiety, developed into panic attacks in my twenties, and then developed into full-blown depression three years after that.

When I was anxious I would have a thought such as, *what if I hurt someone?* Or *I'm not as good as people think I am*. And it would get stuck, I couldn't let it go; so that eventually my head was full of such thoughts and I felt like I would explode.

Do anxious people always get depressed? Are they part of the same thing, like a sliding scale?

Elliot: Someone can suffer from anxiety disorder without also having depression; or suffer from depression without having anxiety disorder. They are distinct illnesses, each with their own diagnosis and symptoms. However, they are closely related, are often experienced together, and there is a lot of crossover in terms of the psychological processes they involve. As a consequence, the psychological therapies with the strongest evidence base – the cognitive behavioural therapies – can have a very similar focus whether they are treating anxiety or depression or both (for example, dealing with avoidance and the worrying and rumination that can be so much a part of these mental illnesses). The medical term for the experience of having more than one illness or condition at a time is 'co-morbidity'.

Jacob: When I was 13 I began getting panic attacks. I had a dismaying dream that started it all, and I woke up freaking out, drenched in sweat, and after that I had panic attacks almost every day. That feeling I woke up with was the same feeling I had when I had my attacks.

They'd happen around two to four times a day. Lying in bed at night they might come more than once. My senses were heightened and there was a ringing in my ears. Every little movement in my toes I felt like I could hear. When the sheets rustled, it sounded like a roar. And if I rolled over it was as if I was in slow motion.

If I get that feeling nowadays I'm always very surprised and it never lasts long. There's no sense of panic when I get it now, it's just a very strange sensation.

I didn't understand what that feeling was, but it was incredibly frightening. Mum took me to the doctor and I was referred to the Kari Centre, which is a community mental health service for teenagers in Auckland. The very first time we went there, these two therapists told me that panic attacks were easy to fix. That day, I just cried and cried. It was probably the built-up terror and then the relief. I couldn't stop. I went there each week and had sessions, and they explained it to me in a really good way and I learnt how to stop the attacks.

But depression . . . I suppose no one can remember the day they got depression. You kind of slide into it, and I just slid into it over the next few months. You feel really low and you can blame it on outside factors, and sometimes for me I got very angry and punched holes in my bedroom wall. I blamed a lot of my feelings on things that were being done to me; that I had to go to school and do things I no longer wanted to do. Sometimes I couldn't get out of bed.

Elliot: There is ongoing research into the relationship between these two illnesses. In the meantime, various studies have revealed the extent to which they co-occur in individuals.

The Dunedin longitudinal study, which is following 1037 people born in 1972 and 1973, acknowledges the 'prevailing notion' that anxiety usually precedes depression for people who experience them both – as it did for JK. However, the opposite can also happen – just as people can get depressed about their anxiety, they can get anxious about their depression. At other times both might just develop together. In the Dunedin longitudinal study, 72 percent of lifetime anxiety cases had a history of depression, and 48 percent of lifetime depression cases had a history of anxiety.

The Christchurch longitudinal study, which over 35 years has studied the progress of a group of 1265 children born in 1977, also found 'a substantial degree of overlap' between the disorders. People with a mood disorder (depression) were six times more likely to get an anxiety disorder than those people who didn't have a mood disorder. Of those who had a mood disorder, 42 percent had a co-morbid anxiety disorder.

The study found that just over one-fifth of young people aged from 16 to 18 met the criteria for a mood disorder, and one-sixth had some form of anxiety disorder. These studies, along with the New Zealand Mental Health Survey, confirm the strength of the relationship between depression and anxiety. And we're not alone with this as findings aren't dissimilar in other parts of the world. It's affecting a lot of our young people, and the earlier we identify and treat it the better.

Hannah (now 19): I think I've always been a pretty anxious person. I wouldn't have recognised that about myself, but when I think back, I was a worrywart, a fingernail biter, a worried person constantly.

My eating disorder started when I'd just turned 15 and went on a school trip overseas for three weeks. I had a couple of panic attacks. I was so anxious I didn't eat for about two weeks, and that was the trigger from there. I remember walking along the street and thinking I had stopped breathing.

I see now that the eating disorder was a manifestation of anxiety.

The way I feel the anxiety in my body is, I can feel it rise up, and I'm not thinking straight. I start fidgeting with everything. But mainly it's the thinking. I get really irrational in my thought processes. And people often say to me, you seem so relaxed. So, outwardly, you wouldn't notice me standing there freaking out, but it's more of an inward manifestation.

I definitely worried about what I looked like and about clothes. We had mufti days at school and I'd literally not be able to go to school on that day.

Schoolwork got more important, everything got more serious. Sport became at rep level not at social level. At the same time, you're supposed to be managing things more by yourself. I think that's where the eating got out of control.

By the time I was in hospital with anorexia, the possibility was raised that I was also suffering from depression. I was terrified. I had anxiety over the idea of having depression. I think it's just the stigma. I was OK having an eating disorder, sort of, but depression was absolutely not OK. It was a label that I understood to mean unstable, unmotivated, weak and unsuccessful. Hopeless. Lonely. Isolated.

I guess what shifted my attitude later on was meeting people who had had depression. I guess I was learning that you can be ill, but that's not who you are; it doesn't define you.

- Depression and anxiety are distinct illnesses, each with their own diagnosis and symptoms.
- They are closely related and are often experienced together, and treatment can be similar.

7.
Teen depression has its own flavour

Kirsty: Depression and anxiety don't look exactly the same in every person, because they are experienced emotionally and physically in an individual's unique context – everyone's story is their own. However, that said, depression does present remarkably similarly for everybody, given how many different contributing factors can be involved.

In particular, it's really important to note that adolescent depression can look different to adult depression. Adult depression is notable for the sadness that's often apparent in the person's feelings. But with teenagers, we might not see the sadness as the predominant feature. We might be more likely to see irritability and aggression – a more reactive, emotional sensitivity – and perhaps some antisocial behaviour. This is one of the reasons that teenage depression can go undiagnosed.

Matt (Levi's new dad): Mental illness sometimes looks like bad behaviour. I used to work as a drug and alcohol counsellor and before that as a school guidance counsellor, and I saw that quite a lot, especially for boys. Depression is completely different for an adolescent male. Depression isn't the signs that you see on TV or that kind of stuff. Sadness: to be sad you have to be completely vulnerable, so what teenage boy is going to allow himself to be that in public? But what is OK in a teenage boy is anger and frustration and aggression, and sometimes violence. I definitely see that. I talk to young people, and throughout the conversation it will turn from 'I'm really pissed off, and so-and-so did this to me' to 'I don't know what's wrong, I just feel really broken.' That kind of thing.

Kirsty: When teenagers get depressed they can easily slide towards drugs and alcohol as a way of escaping from their difficult emotions, and for various other complex reasons to do with their identity and 'fitting in'. It's important that parents, teachers and other caregivers consider that the underlying cause of a teenager's substance abuse might be depression or anxiety; and that 'bad behaviour' in general might indicate underlying mental illness. This is particularly common in boys.

Levi: Teachers have got too much to do to handle kids like me. It's so easy to go, *that kid plays up in class; I'll just send him out.*

The way I see it is, at the verge of destruction, people tend to change, but it's at that exact same point that most people go, *I can't deal with this kid no more.* And *that's* the point where I believe they should do the hard yards and push through, because that's what would knock a brick down from the wall he's put around himself, and then more bricks would come down and that's where you'll have an in.

Elliot: When it comes to diagnosing depression, mental health clinicians generally use the definitions found in the officially recognised diagnostic classification systems. These have a role in defining the different mood disorders. Their purpose is to ensure that anxiety and depression, for example, mean the same thing to different practitioners. They aim to standardise diagnostic practices.

On pages 54–58, there is a summary of the core aspects and symptoms of the main anxiety and depressive disorders, and some other mental disorders where anxiety and depressed mood may be prominent.

There is a wide range of other mental illnesses, too. We have chosen to focus on anxiety and depression because these are by far the most prevalent mental disorders among young people. The World Health Organization estimates that by 2020 depression will be second only to ischaemic heart disease in the amount of disability experienced by sufferers – we call this the 'burden' of disease. Anxiety and depression carry a heavy burden: impaired physical and role functioning, more days in bed due to illness, work days lost, impairment at work and school, and high use of health services. In fact, the disability caused by depression and anxiety is just as great as that caused by common medical conditions such as hypertension, diabetes and arthritis.

- Adolescent depression can look different to adult depression.
- With teenagers, sadness might not be the predominant feature. We might be more likely to see irritability and aggression, particularly so with boys.
- Consider that the underlying cause of a teenager's substance abuse or bad behaviour might be depression or anxiety.

8.
Anxiety – cuddling the fear

Helene: I was a very anxious child, and very shy. I worried about anything and everything. Some things were particularly challenging: speeches, parties, hosting parties. I found it difficult to be the centre of attention. I'd worry that the other kids wouldn't like my party. The funny thing was that the stuff I'd worry about would usually work out quite well, but it didn't stop me worrying the next time around.

I saw shyness as a weakness. I felt so bad about the way I was.

Mostly, I felt guilty that I felt so bad. I knew I had a good life, and my family was (and is) close, well balanced, supportive. I knew that I was very loved. There was no real answer. It made it hard for me to accept.

I certainly didn't know anything about anxiety or depression, and if I did hear anything about them, I thought it was something that happened to older people. I think more awareness is the right thing for young people. Perhaps we don't have to reach rock bottom before we can do something about it. Now I want to tell that child that I was, *it's all OK*. I see all the time and energy that I wasted worrying. It's unbelievable.

I avoided a lot of things I would have liked to do: choir, netball (I'd have such a worry about letting the team down). I did a psychology degree and would like to have been a clinical psychologist, but I'd had such an easy life and felt guilty about the anxiety I had – *what right do I have to feel like this?* If I was to become a psychologist I'd be dealing with people who had serious problems, and they'd look at me and feel, *what does she know?*

I began to train as a teacher, but the trouble for a perfectionist is that teaching doesn't have boundaries. There's always more you can do. I became obsessive about it all – wanting to do a good job and worrying that I wasn't, and that spiralled out of control. I always felt I wasn't good enough, even though I got top marks and was immediately offered a job.

At the end of my training I had a strange summer where I slept and slept. I had no interest in social things. I became obsessive about getting my classroom ready, even though my mentor said, 'You don't need to be trying to create this wonderland in the classroom.'

The school year started and immediately I was not dealing with things. One of the really awful things about the way anxiety manifested for me was that I had these racing, racing thoughts that meant it was very hard to get any perspective. I sat up late making resources, and when I tried to sleep my mind was leaping. I'd been close to the edge before, so I thought I'd be OK this time, too.

Of course my family was concerned and tried to talk to me about it and I'd say, 'It'll come right.' But one day I went down to the supermarket and I was standing in the aisle and I just started to cry. I couldn't stop. By the next morning I felt absolutely sick and I couldn't go to work. I hadn't even made it through the first week of school.

JK: Depression and anxiety are about fear. Raw fear. A series of very, very scary thoughts that are controlling you. It's like being out of control in your head. Fear was a major contributor to my depression; and my anxiety attacks, while they only lasted a few minutes, felt like they lasted three days.

Because fear is so awful, people tend to put fear in the cupboard, all locked away and out of sight: they pretend it isn't there any more. That's what I did. But then the fear gets really pissed off, and when you're not ready it jumps out and attacks you, like a ghost or a scary monster. Now, with my fear, I try and sit it on my knee and give it a cuddle. That brings it closer so that I know it and can identify it; and that takes a lot of the power out of it.

It's a really hard thing to talk about, because every awful situation of fear is different. I can only tell you what works for me. It boils down to being aware of your fear – not in that vague way where it's standing behind you out of sight; not in that way of pushing it away and hoping that bad things won't happen. I mean:

naming it. Really getting to understand it. I'm not saying it's easy – fear is often very complex and hard to grab hold of.

My biggest fear is to do with breaking the family up – coming to New Zealand to follow my career, leaving my daughter Francesca behind, taking the boys out of their familiar setting – and that having long-term effects on my children, which would turn me into a bad parent. I apologised to Niko when he was struggling during the year: 'I'm really sorry,' I told him. He says, 'It's not your fault, you've got to follow your career.' So that's one aspect of the fear I have. But fear is a complex, multi-headed beast, a bit like the three-headed dog in Harry Potter. So I'm worried about my family, but I'm selfish about my career and what I'm trying to achieve.

My fear, from a professional point of view, is probably no different from most people's professional fears: the fear of failing, of feeling I was never good enough to be at the level I want to be at.

So what do I do? If I put all those fears into the cupboard I'll become stressed and I'll start second-guessing. I'll be responding to the wrong things; I'll be acting on false information. So instead, I get close to the fears. I try and break them into little pieces so I can see them better, rather than keeping them as one big feeling of fear – and I talk to the people who they affect. I keep addressing my doubts and fears. I work on those insecurities. I call it 'cuddling the fear'.

Fear is an emotion, just like love is. So if you were to try and take the fear out of fear, what would you do to it? Most fear is associated with hiding, shaking, running away from a situation. It's a black thing, a devil type of image, and we want to get away from it. The last thing that ugly creature wants is a cuddle. So grab hold of it and give it a cuddle – this breaks it down a wee bit and takes the fear out of it. If you can address and understand your fears, communicate them to the people who matter, and then 'cuddle' those fears, you take away some of their power. It's like laughing in the face of fear.

When I was depressed, my fear was a constant thing, a physical and emotional nightmare. It had so much power over me that it was like a black hole, sucking the life out of me. I don't experience fear like that any more, and that's because I don't lock it away where it can grow in the dark.

I live a very public life. I think that, when I was younger, that was behind some of the confusion I felt – I had a lot of fear, but I did my best to ignore it. I knew my life looked great, but I felt there was this huge gap between the way people saw me and the way I was. But when you bare your soul – as I have done very publicly – life in public becomes a little bit easier. Now I have the ability to be honest and open about what I'm feeling or what I'm doing. There's no real difference between my public image and who I am. There are no secrets about the kind of person I am, and that's good for me because it's in secrets – in that cupboard – that fear takes root and grows.

Living so publicly doesn't affect the scale of my fears. It doesn't make me more afraid of failing. Failure is failure. Newspaper articles speculate all the time about failure, about expectations. That's just the way it goes; and I knew that when I came back to live in New Zealand. But I don't have failure any more in my life: I just have *having a go* or *not having a go*. Do I want to succeed? Hell, yes. I want to win the competition. Some things are in my control; some things are out of my control. But if it doesn't work and I'm not good enough, my success has been that I had a go.

Elliot: Naming the fear – and through this identifying it as something external to who you are – and then approaching it, is probably the most important part of the cognitive behavioural therapies for anxiety and depression.

When we avoid, nothing changes. When we allow ourselves to experience painful emotions and take a good look at them, we learn that the distressing feeling is just a feeling – it's tolerable and can't harm us. With that learning, confidence increases and we become even more comfortable approaching our fears.

One process going on here is *habituation*, where the trigger for the fear no longer prompts fear. The other process is the development of *mindfulness* – the ability to spot negative emotions, observe them, and let them go, rather than be carried away by them.

- Anxiety can cause people to avoid things and miss opportunities.
- Fear is a big part of the experience of both anxiety and depression.
- In JK's experience, which is a common one, pretending the fear wasn't there was disastrous.
- It's much better to acknowledge the fear, and name it – this helps to overcome it.

9.
What are depressive and anxiety disorders?

Depressive disorders

When people talk about depression, they are generally referring to the diagnosis of 'major depressive disorder'. This is just one of a number of conditions grouped within a broader category of 'depressive disorders'. These are all marked by low or irritable mood, along with physical symptoms and changes in thinking that make it difficult for people to function in their lives. The two main depressive disorders are 'major depressive disorder' and 'dysthymia'.

Major depressive disorder involves depressive episodes that last at least two weeks – and almost always much longer. These episodes involve some combination of the following symptoms: depressed or irritable mood, a lack of interest in things that are normally enjoyed, weight and/or appetite changes, increases or reductions in sleep, physical agitation or slowing, loss of energy, concentration difficulties, and thoughts of death (which can include suicidal thoughts).

Dysthymia (or persistent depressive disorder) is a longer-term depression, where symptoms are present for at least a year (in adolescents) or two (in adults).

Grief is something that can also look very much like depression, but is generally considered a normal life experience rather than an illness. However, grief can fail to resolve for some people within normal timeframes, or the loss that triggers the grief may also trigger depression, so it is important to seek professional advice where a grief response appears out of proportion within the culture where this occurs.

Anxiety disorders

What anxiety disorders all have in common is disproportionate levels of fear and anxiety that impact on people's behaviour and have a very disruptive effect on their lives. Common to most anxiety states is an overestimation of danger, and an underestimation of the ability to cope.

The fear and anxiety are often accompanied by the 'fight or flight' response. This is an adaptation humans have developed in which our nervous systems become aroused in order to help us fight or flee what we think is dangerous. Typical aspects of the fight or flight response include increased breathing and heart rate, sweating, and muscles becoming tense. Other physical symptoms that can follow from the fight or flight response include nausea, shaking, and paling or flushing. The particular fears and associated symptoms of anxiety often then lead to avoidance of the situation or thing that is associated with the fear, even though the fear is unwarranted.

The following are common anxiety disorders.

Panic disorder is diagnosed when people struggle with recurrent panic attacks, some of which are experienced as occurring without any obvious trigger – 'out of the blue'. People who have panic disorder tend to worry that the anxiety symptoms they experience during panic are signs of serious physical health problems, such as heart or brain conditions. They may also worry that they will be embarrassed if others see them panicking.

Specific phobia involves disproportionate fear and anxiety about specific situations or objects that the sufferer actively avoids or only tolerates with distress. Common categories that are a focus for specific phobias include animals (e.g. spiders or dogs); the natural environment (e.g. heights or water); and blood, needles or medical procedures. It is not uncommon for people diagnosed with specific phobia to have concerns about more than one of these objects or situations.

In **social anxiety disorder** (social phobia) the focus of the anxiety relates to the fear of being seen to be anxious and then being judged negatively by other people. Situations that are avoided, or only tolerated with great distress, tend to involve social interactions (e.g. meeting and talking to new people), being watched (e.g. when eating), or performing in the presence of other people (e.g. public speaking).

Generalised anxiety disorder involves prolonged (at least six months) disproportionate worry and anxiety over a broad range of concerns. Typically these might cover work, health, family and relationships, along with more mundane day-to-day issues. In teens the focus of worry may be on doubts about their competence or abilities. The worry is experienced as very difficult to control, and is accompanied by a range of physical, behavioural and cognitive symptoms of anxiety.

Agoraphobia is anxiety triggered by being in particular situations, typically on public transport, in open spaces (e.g. markets), in enclosed spaces (e.g. shops), in crowds, or being alone away from home. People with agoraphobia fear that something terrible will happen; often they fear they will become incapacitated or humiliated by their anxiety, and that they will not be able to escape the situation – or at least not without great difficulty. As a consequence, the feared situation is actively avoided, or only tolerated with great distress.

As well as these common anxiety disorders it is important to mention panic attacks. *Panic attacks* are rapidly developing episodes of acute fear and dread (involving the fight or flight symptoms mentioned earlier) that usually last just a few minutes. However, they can recur so quickly that multiple panic attacks can be perceived as a single, longer episode.

People can have panic attacks without having a depressive or anxiety disorder. However, panic attacks are sometimes experienced by people with depression, and (more frequently) by people with a range of different anxiety disorders.

Other disorders in which anxiety or depressed mood may be prominent

Obsessive-compulsive disorder (OCD) is characterised by obsessive thoughts that cause anxiety, and compulsive behaviours or thoughts that are engaged in to relieve that anxiety. The obsessions include unwanted thoughts (e.g. about being dirty or contaminated) or urges (e.g. sexual). The compulsions will match these (e.g. hand-washing to decontaminate, or praying to atone for thoughts experienced as 'improper'). The obsessions and compulsions are so time-consuming – they may take hours each day – that they cause disruption in the person's life.

Post-traumatic stress disorder (PTSD) involves the experience of distress (including anxiety) in response to reminders of a traumatic event (e.g. an actual or threatened death, injury or violence). These reminders can take the form of 're-experiencing' the trauma in memories, dreams or 'flashbacks' in which someone feels like they are reliving the event. Things (e.g. people and places) that are associated with the trauma are actively avoided in an attempt to manage anxiety. Like OCD, PTSD has long been classed as an anxiety disorder in some classification systems.

Eating disorders all involve some disturbance of eating, or behaviour around eating, resulting in physical health problems or other disabling problems. The most common eating disorders are anorexia nervosa and bulimia nervosa.

Anorexia is marked by restricted eating resulting in abnormally low body weight, which is associated with fear or anxiety about putting on weight or being fat, and impaired perceptions of body shape or weight.

Bulimia involves episodes of overeating (binge eating) that are experienced as 'out of control', and which are followed by anxiety-driven attempts to prevent gaining weight, such as self-induced vomiting, use of laxatives, or excessive exercise.

Adjustment disorder can be diagnosed when people develop strong and disproportionate emotional reactions (that can include anxiety) in response to other, not necessarily traumatic, stressful events (e.g. a change in schools).

Bipolar disorders include periods of depression and periods of 'mania', involving unusually elevated mood, activity and energy.

Schizophrenia and other psychotic disorders

Psychotic disorders are serious conditions characterised by delusions (fixed false beliefs), hallucinations (false perceptions, e.g. of hearing or seeing things), disorganised thinking and behaviour (reflected in speech that is hard to follow and difficulties with goal directed behaviour), and so-called 'negative symptoms' (reductions in emotional expression, motivation, social interest, and talkativeness). The course of these conditions can include episodes of depression.

Diagnosing a mental disorder requires ruling out physical health conditions, the effects of a physical health condition, and the effects of a substance such as a drug or alcohol. All three of these may produce depressive or anxiety symptoms or states that look like a mental disorder. It is therefore essential that a medical practitioner rules out those possibilities before the diagnosis of a mental disorder such as depression or anxiety can be made.

There is considerable debate among mental health professionals about these systems of psychiatric classifications. However, they have their place in helping clinicians diagnose the clusters of symptoms an individual might have and what treatments to use.

For more information on mental health disorders in youth, see the websites in the Resources section at the back of the book.

10.
On the spectrum of 'human'

Kirsty: What's interesting about the painful thoughts and negative mood states that come with anxiety and depression is that most people experience those to a certain degree at some time or another. We all have concerns and doubts about ourselves, the world we live in and our futures. To an extent these concerns and associated emotions are a part of being human; and they crop up throughout anyone's life, including during adolescence.

Unfortunately, when we become unwell we can get stuck on these natural questions and experiences. They grow in significance, torment us, consume our head space and our time, and start to impact negatively on our lives. We can't just 'move on' from these thoughts, 'dismiss them' or distract ourselves from them as we may have done previously.

Because the depressive and anxiety disorders are so closely related to ordinary human experience, some of the ways of treating them are not so different from learning how to live a full and healthy life. Similar psychological principles that are used to treat mental illness can be applied to human thriving. The field of positive psychology has developed around these ideas.

I find I use lots of psychology principles and strategies within my own life when I have struggles or challenging things to do. These might include identifying and challenging the way I might be thinking about a situation; learning to accept and sit with difficult emotions; and setting myself goals with small identifiable steps and supports and rewards that keep me going. There are additional strategies that we will talk about later in the book, relating to cultivating resilience.

Ironically, recovering from mental illness can be resilience-building in itself. This is through the experience of what is called post-traumatic growth. People who have worked through depression or anxiety, and who have worked through the therapy, often find themselves in a stronger and more 'well' position at the end of it than before they became ill. This is because they have developed a sense of strength from having coped with a major challenge, have increased empathy for others' suffering, and a greater sense of connection because of this; a greater sense of perspective and an appreciation of what is important to them in life; and potentially even some spiritual change associated with having a greater sense of purpose or meaning in life.

JK: That is so true for me. Post-traumatic growth describes my personal journey. Depression was 'traumatic' – it totally shook my foundations. But 'growth' describes what I've been about ever since. Since depression, my whole philosophy has been about continual personal growth. That's what keeps me well.

- Many of the emotions and worries inherent in depression and anxiety are a natural part of being human, but are taken to extremes where people get stuck on them.
- Some of the psychological principles used in treatments for depression and anxiety can be applied within strategies for living a full life beyond recovery from illness.
- Recovering from illness in itself can help move people toward the healthy end of the psychological spectrum of being human.

11.
My brain just won't work

JK: When I was depressed I had the classic symptoms that I now know were because of the effect of the illness on my brain. I couldn't cope with thinking, couldn't remember anything, not even what happened 10 minutes ago. I felt like my mind was shrinking because I had to concentrate so hard on getting through the minute, through the day. You're not thinking, 'It's sunny outside' – your world has become very narrow. The biggest thing it took away from me was my confidence.

Elliot: Most people are aware that depression involves low mood. However, people who experience depression often also struggle to make sense of the difficulties they have with cognitive functioning, such as concentration, making decisions (even insignificant ones), planning, and remembering things – which are also symptoms of depression. For many people, these symptoms can be some of the most distressing. This aspect of depression is often closely linked with the key factor that determines when low mood crosses into clinical depression – the negative impact on a person's day-to-day functioning. It is very hard to operate in any role that requires clear thinking when you're depressed. This often plays out at work for adults, whereas for teens it is obviously more likely to show up in a lowering of academic performance at school. The good news is that effective treatment of depression – psychological or medical – can turn around those thinking difficulties.

JK also mentioned the other way depression can affect thinking – that is, the 'style' of a person's thinking. By this, we mean the negative, pessimistic conclusions and attitudes that people often develop when unwell with depression.

One of the nasty things about depression is that these thinking problems (and other symptoms) often work together to keep the condition going. You can't think clearly, so you give yourself a hard time about that, so your thinking becomes very negative. This leads to your mood and confidence dropping, so you start to withdraw from people, your life lacks stimulation, and you become preoccupied with your situation and distracted by negative thoughts – and so your concentration may get worse! The good news is that the vicious cycles that maintain depression (and anxiety) can be broken by effective medical and psychological treatments. These treatments are designed to target those 'maintaining' factors – the symptoms themselves, and the unhelpful behaviours we engage in to cope with them.

- People with depression may have difficulty with cognitive functioning, so can experience problems with remembering things, making decisions, planning, setting priorities and taking action.
- Medication and/or psychotherapy can overcome these symptoms.

12.
Warning signs – when to worry

Benson: If I had a tough time I think I'd probably go a bit quiet, and a bit like not paying attention.

Adam: I'd be quiet, too. I'd probably spend more time alone.

Moana: But being alone and being productive is different to being alone and curled up in a ball and crying. I like to be alone to read. I don't think that's an alarming signal.

Olivia: I'd get angry quickly.

Ellen: With kids, staying in their bedroom is probably a sign. Like, if they don't come out.

Anish: I had a friend who got depression. He was quiet. He pretty much withdrew himself away from everyone else. He sat by himself, kind of isolating himself. He didn't work. Half the time he'd just sleep in class.

Scarlet: One friend started to lose motivation quite quickly for things that she was usually really good at. She wagged school sometimes. The biggest thing we noticed was she either left class early or didn't come to school. It was just really out of character.

JK: I wonder a lot about warning signs. I wonder whether me getting homesick in Hunua was a sign that I was going to develop anxiety later on, or just a normal part of being a kid. I wonder about my own kids – if they're nervous about exams at 13, is that an indication of anxiety? How can we know, and how can we parent so that those early signs – if that's what they are – don't ever have to turn into an illness?

The first step has got to be: knowing our kids, and being aware of what's going on for them. Knowing what to watch out for. Staying alert. Knowing what's normal for them, so that we can tell when things are changing and the danger bells are ringing.

There wasn't a lot of psychology when I was growing up. It was a different era. I don't think people put a lot of thought into parenting in those days, not in a psychological sense. Society was just assumed to be banging everyone into shape. We'd go out on the street, play with our mates, there was much more community. There were 10 kids in our street and we all grew up together, and the parenting was different.

Nowadays, someone like me might have been parented a bit differently, perhaps. I was shy. Shy to the point of ridiculous, probably lacking a bit of self-esteem, and underachieving at school. My innate character was I was never quite good enough. I wasn't too worried about the future, but I wasn't really striving as much as I should have. My shyness meant I avoided things. So many things that I can't even think of them all – parties, all sorts of things. When I was 14, I won a rugby prize that was to be presented at an event by the great rugby league player Mark Graham, who was actually a cousin of mine. I refused to go because I was too shy to stand up in front of other people. I hid behind not talking and being shy.

Maybe those things were just part of growing up. As adolescents grow up, there can be a lack of self-esteem as they look for their place in the world, and it's really important to know how to parent for that – to be sensitive about it, and not dismissive, but not panic-stricken, either.

But did my shyness and lack of self-esteem help me get depressed? Was it part of the mix?

I do know that when I made it into the All Blacks at 19, I learnt very quickly what people were expecting and I gave them that. I faked it. I created another persona. It was all just acting. But because I'd never dealt with those childhood feelings, they were still all there, and the gap grew between my public persona and what was still going on inside.

I think a lot of good things are going on these days, as far as our awareness of other people's feelings goes, and our attitude to getting help. Generally, we're a lot more sensitive to what's going on, and that's great.

Elliot: I agree with JK's point that staying alert and connected is the big thing for parents. If we really know our kids, we'll be far more likely to notice when things go wrong – and that comes down to listening to our own gut feelings, as well.

It's human nature to want everything to be normal: we don't want difficulty and disruption. But this desire to avoid potential conflict and drama alongside our busy way of life can cause us to look away for too long when an adolescent is developing a mental illness. It's all too easy to convince ourselves that 'she'll be right', because we know how hard it's going to be to stare at this problem head-on. We are afraid of overreacting, afraid of having to make hard decisions, afraid of the conflict that may well arise. But the risks of not taking action are great.

Adrienne (Marly's mum): In the months leading up to her crash, Marly didn't talk happily about anything any more. Everything was a bit harder, and everything was a bit more miserable. She talked about school and her friends as if it was just a bit harder, instead of being this great place. I'd find her crying in her bedroom, and I'd say, 'What are you crying about?' There'd always be some minor adolescent thing, but none of it seemed enough to explain it, really. Or she'd say, 'I don't know' or 'Go away, Mum, you don't understand.' She was irritable. She didn't sleep well. But she'd never been a great sleeper, so I didn't really take that much notice.

She wasn't badgering me to go and see friends. She ate a lot of junk food, and was putting on weight, but how do you know? She maintained her schoolwork, but it took her longer and it was harder and she worried over it. It was taking her a long time.

We didn't act. That's my only regret, and it's quite a significant regret – a big learning.

Elliot: It's not easy, to be sure. For adolescents, the symptoms might come and go over time. Also, as psychiatrist David Fassler points out in *Help Me, I'm Sad*, kids aren't always sophisticated enough, don't always have the language, to say things like: 'I feel like there's no hope left.' Instead, they might pick fights at school, or get frequent tummyaches and not want to go to school, or even begin to experiment with drugs and alcohol.

For parents, then, the thing to watch out for is change: a change in behaviour, a change in attitude.

Kirsty: First, we have to get to know our well child so that we are sensitive to what's going on for them and can detect when the way they are thinking and behaving is different to what it was before, when they are 'unwell'. It's a bit like being an investigator – and that's something most parents get pretty good at! Learn about symptoms and signs. And don't be afraid to trust your gut instinct and seek help if you are worried. (There's a lot more about this later on.)

When things are changing anyway, as your young person navigates adolescence and experiments with their identity, noticing unhealthy or worrying change is challenging. It can also be useful to consider the following.

- Is the change *persistent* – that is, do the problems never really go away? There's a difference between the child who is grumpy, irritable, sad and withdrawn for a day or so but then gets back to normal activities, and the child for whom these moods are ongoing or intense for a couple of weeks, go away for a short time but then come back again.
- Is the change *pervasive* – that is, does it cover a whole lot of areas? For example is your young person sad and withdrawn at school, home and socially, or are they just withdrawing more at home as they negotiate the changes in their relationship with you?
- Because some of the symptoms are very like normal adolescent behaviour, the key is to look for the *combination* of symptoms. If your teen has stopped paying much attention to their personal hygiene, that in itself might not indicate a mental illness; but if it's combined with other things, such as a noticeable lack of self-esteem, difficulty concentrating and a failure to go to usual sports practice – and these things are not

just a short-term response to a sad event such as a relationship break-up – then they could indicate a problem.
- Is the change *different* from their peers? Is your teen changing to fit in with their peers, or are they actually becoming more distant from their peers?
- Finally, an important question to ask is: What *impact* are these changes you're seeing – the 'symptoms' – having on their daily functioning? It's a tricky thing: we're talking about so-called signs and symptoms that are not medical (like a high temperature), yet we're calling it an illness. But really, if the changes are signs of an illness, they will have an impact on how well the adolescent is functioning.

Janet (Helene's mum): Looking back, I think that Helene's depression was brought on by her perfectionism. It created so much anxiety and stress, and eventually led to a state of sheer exhaustion. There was a build-up over a long period of time, starting when she was in primary school. Even from a young age, she would drive herself to the limit in the need to have her work absolutely perfect. If something wasn't 'right' in her eyes, she would tear it up and start it all over again.

These times were extremely hard for me to cope with, not knowing how to help her and when (if at all) to intervene. I would try to convince her that her work was fine the way it was and to stop worrying, but she wouldn't be able to rest until it was done to her standard. She would get more anxious and sometimes even angry if she thought we were trying to stop her. It was hard to know whether to take her at her word and just support her, or whether some stronger action was needed. In the end I just had to be there to comfort her through the trials and upsets that came with this. I hoped that as she got older she would learn to deal with it and not push herself so hard.

At the time there was very little information out there about mental health, especially in children.

Kirsty: The change can be more difficult to note in someone for whom it doesn't occur suddenly – where it's a gradual thing. That more gradual depression is harder to pick, so it's important to note that while, for some, the change might be quite marked and easily picked up by school and by family, for others it's slower.

So, if you have a sneaking, gut feeling that things have shifted for your child and that something is wrong, but you don't want to make a fuss or label them, my first thought would be: trust your gut. You're the parent. And with a child who is experiencing depression or anxiety, where there's a hopelessness or a fearfulness and they can't quite express what's going on, they need you to be putting out the feelers for them.

Lyndy Matthews (psychiatrist): Trust your instincts and don't make assumptions. Don't assume that because your teen's demeanour, temperament or behaviour changes it's *because he's an adolescent* or *because she's hormonal*. I don't think adolescents are these magical beasts who are so different from us. They're actually small, slightly younger humans. Yes, they're more volatile. Yes, their brains are still developing. Yes, their judgments aren't always great. But if they are developing mood and behaviour changes that you would be concerned about if they were 22, allow yourself to be concerned even if they're in their teens. Consider that your child might need some help with their mental health. Consider that first.

Claire (Julia's mum): Things that she would usually get excited about weren't exciting her. She wanted to be in her room a lot, and she was very emotional. She had no friends.

Because Julia was depressed she lost her zeal. She has always liked to do things well, and as a young child would get a lot of joy from her art and music and schoolwork. But she was in a dark place where there was no enjoyment any more; it was all about doing it well, about being perfect and getting it right. Trying to do things perfectly. Art projects that were supposed to take three-quarters of an hour of homework were taking her five hours. The thing she was good at, she would say, 'It's not good enough.' She became inward-looking, darker, focused on that dark inward place.

When you're happy, you do these things and feel that sense of achievement. But the negative voices were getting strong in her head.

- Stay connected to your kids so you'll be far more likely to notice when things go wrong.
- The thing to watch out for is change: a change in behaviour; a change in attitude.
- If you have a feeling things aren't quite right for your child – trust your gut instinct. A child experiencing depression probably can't quite express what's going on, and they need you to be putting out the feelers for them.

Signs and symptoms of depression to be alert for in adolescents

Emotions

- sad, depressed, miserable or irritable mood a lot of the time (more easily tearful, upset or reactive)

Physical signs

- agitated, restless, on edge or slowed down, lacking in energy
- changes in appetite – significant weight loss or gain, or failure to put on weight to match growth
- sleeping changes – difficulty sleeping, or sleeping a lot
- loss of energy and feeling tired all the time
- difficulty concentrating – changes in how they're doing at school, difficulty starting or finishing schoolwork
- expressing aches and pains, such as headache or stomach ache, that don't have a medical basis

Behaviours

- loss of interest in activities that were previously enjoyed (beyond just growing out of activities)
- not looking after appearance
- withdrawal – avoiding friends, family, pulling back from seeing friends
- increase in alcohol or drug use to manage emotions

Thinking

- feeling worthless or guilty – making critical or blaming comments about self
- describing feeling overwhelmed; lacking confidence to make decisions
- having thoughts of death or suicide or feeling hopeless (*what's the point, I'm a failure, life's not worth living*)

Key things for you to consider

- Has there been a change (gradual or sudden)? Is it very different from what they were like previously or what their peers are like?
- Is the change persistent? Has it been around for quite some time, or if it goes away does it keep coming back?
- Is it occurring across multiple settings (e.g. home, school, social contexts)?
- Is the change impacting negatively on their daily life – at school; in friendships, family and other relationships; at sports?

Signs and symptoms of anxiety to be alert for in adolescents

Emotions

- feeling on edge, 'worried' or tense most of the time
- constant dread that something bad is going to happen
- intense, overwhelming or excessive fears
- irritability

Physical signs

- racing heart, sweaty, tingling, shaking, dizziness, shortness of breath
- nausea or stomach aches
- difficulty concentrating; forgetting things
- feeling detached
- difficulty sleeping because of worrying thoughts

Behaviours

- avoidance of situations, people or places that are associated with the anxiety
- overwhelming urges to perform rituals (physical or mental) that relieve the anxiety
- perfectionism, holding very high standards and being overly responsible

Thinking

- uncontrollable or overwhelming panic
- ongoing intense, negative, anxious thoughts that others may describe as 'silly' or out of proportion (e.g. *I'm going crazy, I'm having a heart attack, what if . . .?*)

Key things for you to consider

Different combinations of symptoms can indicate different types of anxiety disorders (see the section on anxiety disorders in chapter 9).

- Is this out of proportion for the circumstances and for their developmental stage?
- Do they respond to reassurance, or do symptoms continue and increase over time?
- Is it impacting negatively on their daily life – school, sport, friendships, family and other relationships?

See thelowdown.co.nz and youthbeyondblue.com for more detailed information about depression and anxiety and their symptoms.

13.
Why am I like this?

JK: People would say to me, 'What have you got to be depressed about? You're an All Black, you've got a car sponsor, you travel all over the world.' So I would just close right down and go into myself and wouldn't talk to anyone, because I thought it was a weakness, not an illness.

I spent years looking for reasons – *why am I like this?* But in the end it was irrelevant. Looking for reasons hindered me from getting well. The day I accepted it as an illness – that is, something without blame – was the day I overcame it and started getting well.

Lyndy Matthews (psychiatrist): We can always make up a story to explain the symptoms of depression, without actually naming it as an illness: she failed her exam; his relationship broke up. It seems quite valid, although what they're doing is naming stresses and circumstances. But there's a point at which a person slides from wellness into depression or a significant anxiety disorder, and once they've crossed that line they are much less likely to be able to put it into words and to ask for help. Depression is very sneaky and very insidious, and people are in it before they realise it.

Elliot: Do you remember how, in *All Blacks Don't Cry*, I told JK about the 'Four Ps'? I'm going to touch on them again, as it's a useful framework for understanding why an individual's particular mood or anxiety disorder may have developed and, more importantly, for identifying strengths and targeting treatment. The Four Ps are:

Predisposing factors – any background factors that can increase risk for depression or anxiety (things in your background such as a family history of mental health issues, and also things in the young person's environment or background such as abuse of some kind).

Precipitating factors – why this is happening now (what is currently going on that has unsettled or stressed the young person).

Perpetuating factors – what is keeping it going (things that maintain the illness, such as drug and alcohol abuse, loneliness and other stressful life events).

Protective factors – what can help the young person (the strengths within the young person and their family or community that could help them become well again).

When a young person becomes unwell, it's natural to wonder what 'caused' it. The answer is likely to comprise a range of factors – biological, environmental and psychological. Each factor might increase the risk of a person experiencing depression; but no single factor determines that this particular person will experience depression at this time.

There is clearly a genetic factor in depression and anxiety: young people whose relatives suffer from depression are more vulnerable. Children whose parents have depression are six times more likely to have depression themselves. Studies of identical and non-identical twins show that genetics accounts for 40 percent of the risk, and environmental effects account for the other 60 percent.

Interestingly, the Dunedin longitudinal study showed that children with a short form of a particular gene, and who were maltreated as children (that is, experienced physical abuse, sexual abuse, or who had harsh or rejecting parents), have a high likelihood of developing depressive disorder as adults; while those who do not have this short form of the gene have a low likelihood of depression, even if they were maltreated as children.

This is a difficult area. In some ways it's very good for people to know that there is this genetic, physical component to depression – it certainly supports the fact that depression and anxiety are illnesses, and not to do with, for instance, a lack of willpower. The knowledge of family history can act as a warning sign, giving you a chance to take preventive steps.

However, it's also true that having a genetic tendency does not mean that any individual *will* develop depression. And this is where the really good news comes in: with the right kind of support, a child can become the kind of problem-solving individual who is less likely to fall into the negative thinking patterns that comprise depression.

Resilience. If we can learn to be more resilient we can actually prevent depression and anxiety becoming problematic in a young person's life. We will look into this in depth in a later chapter.

As parents, it's so easy to blame ourselves for everything that goes wrong in our child's life. Guilt! Parents often say, 'If there's anything to feel guilty about, I'll find it!' There is no blame in depression, because the nature of it – the causes – are so complex. However, there are things we can do to help our children become well; and there are things we can do to help prevent mental illness in the first place.

It's not your fault. Mental illness is caused by the interaction between genetics, brain chemistry, and stressful events and relationships (and we all have stressful events in our lives – it's part of being human). The cumulative effect of these factors contributes to a person's vulnerability: the more risk factors there are interacting, the greater a person's vulnerability. However, all those factors are also interacting with the person's protective factors, so that someone with a high number of risk factors but also a high number of protective factors may be less likely to develop depression, or to have it for a shorter time.

- There is clearly a genetic factor in depression, and young people whose relatives suffer from depression are more vulnerable.
- A genetic tendency does not mean that any individual *will* develop depression.
- Mental illness is caused by the interaction between genetics, brain chemistry, and stressful events and relationships.
- Alongside risk factors that may predispose someone to anxiety or depression, people have protective factors – such as coping strategies or other resources that reduce the risk of becoming unwell.
- Our parenting approach can be a protective factor. There are things we can do to help our children become well, and there are things we can do to help prevent mental illness occurring in the first place.

14.
Biology is not destiny

JK: No one had told me that one of my aunts was locked up in Kingseat (a former psychiatric hospital) for six weeks. Then I got mental illness. Now I know there's a genetic aspect to it, I want to know how to identify in my kids any possible anxiety or tendency to get depressed. What do I do as a parent?

Hannah: Dad suffered from depression. I think it would have been good to have had a conversation about Dad's journey, probably when I was about 11 and my own anxiety was showing itself a bit more. Just hearing what Dad had gone through would have been helpful. I look at him now and he's a great dad and a really successful businessman, and hearing how he'd come through this crazy stuff would have been good.

I can remember once I made one of those glib throwaway remarks: 'I nearly had a panic attack.' Of course it was a huge exaggeration, and Mum said, 'That's not appropriate to say, it's a really serious thing.' At the time I thought, *how annoying, everyone says that*. But now I think that might have been a good opportunity for us to have a proper talk about everything – because I knew nothing about anxiety or mental illness at all.

I guess a lot of adults might just kind of hope that if they ignore it, it will go away – but the worst-case scenario is what happens if you do nothing.

I wonder if they thought that telling us might jinx us or spread it; or that maybe we'd label ourselves. So my message to parents would be: don't be scared to take it seriously, to dig a bit deeper. The worst thing that can happen is that you'll get a diagnosis of something that's unfortunate but entirely manageable and treatable.

Elliot: There's no doubt that anxiety and depression run in families – just as in some families there is a strong history of bowel cancer or diabetes. The Australian psychologist Ronald Rapee, in his book on childhood anxiety, *Helping Your Anxious Child*, puts it like this (and everything he says can be applied to a child suffering from depression, too):

> Research has shown that what is passed on from parent to child is not a specific tendency to be shy or to worry about the dark, but a general personality that is more emotionally sensitive than other people's. Just as people vary in how tall they are or the colour of their hair, people vary in how generally emotional they are. Anxious children tend to have a personality that is more emotional than the average. A large part of this is due to their genes. On the positive side, this means that they are likely to be more caring, kind, honest and loving. But on the negative side, this emotionality means that they are more likely to worry, brood, feel down and be fearful.

So, having a family history of depression or anxiety is a predisposing factor. And onto that side of the scales we must also put 'parent modelling'. Children sometimes copy their parents – they copy our way of coping with the world. If you are depressed or anxious and you cope by avoiding or withdrawing from situations, for instance, there's a good chance your child might learn to do the same. On the other hand, if you model healthy ways of coping such as problem-solving or asking for help, they'll learn those, too.

Kirsty: If you have suffered from depression yourself, your child's chances of developing the illness are greater. If you and the child's other parent have both experienced depression, your child's chances are greater again. It's definitely something to be aware of and to watch out for.

We need to remember, however, that biology is not destiny. Parents can understandably get really worried about genetics – they remember their own experiences with depression, or their parents';

or they may have very distressing memories of a particular aunt or grandparent whose whole life was determined and severely limited by mental illness. When a child begins to display symptoms that remind them of these earlier family examples, it can set off denial – it's just too awful to think about – and so they either ignore it and hope it will go away, or they become overanxious.

The thing is, though, that it won't be the same for your child as it was for you or older members of your family. Things have moved on; times have changed. So much more is known now about mental illness, and treatments are more effective. Treatments are available now that were not available even a generation ago, and there is good self-help material available. We've still got a way to go, but there are a lot more options and support available.

The other thing to remember is that genetic vulnerability isn't the only thing that gets passed on. JK worries about his kids inheriting his tendency to anxiety and depression – but his kids are also inheriting his strengths, and all the knowledge that he's gained through his experiences. JK has an awareness – he knows what it has been like for him, and he's alert to depression and anxiety. He's developed strategies and things that keep him well. These are positives he can pass on to his kids. They can be protective factors as well.

These sorts of things can help a parent be more aware, and act quickly and early so that their child has the best chance of prevention or recovery, and a well life.

- A family history of depression or anxiety is a predisposing factor, but biology is not destiny.
- There have been significant developments in our knowledge and treatment of mental health issues.
- Kids can inherit genetics and personality styles.
- Kids can also inherit knowledge, awareness and positive ways of coping.

15.
The risks

Hayley: Before everything bad happened, I was one of those kids who was happy and had lots of friends. I was really young, not a care in the world. Innocence! But we moved houses when I was eight and I went to a new school, and later that year my parents split and my mum left. For some reason kids started picking on me for that: 'Ha ha, you've got no mum!' I was the new kid so I didn't have friends who might have protected me. It's easy to pick on a new kid.

I was sad all the time, and I always blamed myself. I couldn't concentrate in class. My grades weren't very good, so I was bullied about being dumb – just anything they could find.

I didn't get any support. Dad had a lot on his plate, looking after three kids. He didn't see what was happening to me. One of my teachers at least did know what had happened with my mum, because one day when I got really upset I must have mentioned it and she was like, 'That's not an excuse.' Because I was young I didn't even think about talking to anyone about stuff like that.

When I look back now, I see a little child who was really unhappy. I used to sit alone. The other kids would have thought, *we're going to get picked on if we hang out with her.* I basically sat in my classroom every break and read books.

I was left out of everything – always the one picked last, like you see in movies.

Elliot: This might sound a bit circular, but one of the biggest predisposing factors or risks for your child is previous depression. This is a big one. Research indicates that if a child has had an episode of depression before the age of 18, they have around a 40 percent chance of having another episode before their mid-twenties. So, having had depression is a significant predictor for getting depression again. This is why it is so important to diagnose and treat depression as soon as possible, because when it is treated effectively the risk of recurrence is significantly reduced. Children – just like adults – can learn to recognise the warning signals and take positive steps before it becomes overwhelming. This is particularly the case where an adolescent has had a psychological therapy that includes the learning of healthy coping strategies and a relapse-prevention component.

As Hayley's story highlights, stressful life events are also really significant and insinuate themselves into the mix as predisposing factors, precipitating (trigger) factors and perpetuating (maintaining) factors. For children and teens, obvious stressors are: parents at conflict, separating and divorcing; death of a parent; changing schools; pregnancy; becoming involved in drugs and alcohol. Yet not all children who experience a traumatic event will go on to develop an anxiety or mood disorder. As we mentioned before, it's the number of risk factors and the interaction between them that make someone vulnerable. Let's go through some of the key risk factors.

Abuse – whether it's sexual, physical or psychological – can increase risk for a mental disorder. The Christchurch longitudinal study found the likelihood of mental disorder – including anxiety, depression, substance dependence and suicide – was 2.4 times higher for those who had experienced sexual abuse, and 1.5 times higher for physical abuse. Abuse can lead a child to believe that they are worthless. And as is apparent from Levi's story, this can be seen in pent-up rage and despair that can change the child, in turn, into either a bully or a passive 'victim'.

Levi: My relatives beat me every day, and told me how I was ugly and my laugh was ugly. I was scared all the time, and after they went to sleep at night I'd sneak outside and lie on our driveway and cry. And this might be a bit weird, but there's this star up in the sky, the brightest star in the sky, and I used to stare at it and cry to my mum because I wanted my mum back.

I didn't know she'd let me go. As a kid I never knew. I thought they just took me from my mum.

When I was about nine I discovered fighting. A bigger boy was picking on my friend and something snapped inside me, and I got up and all the anger was right there and I went for gold on that guy. All this anger. It felt good. I got really evil. I'd get smashed, but then go back the next day and smash them. I remember laughing. I like this, I like hurting people, I like this.

Things got worse at home, until one night I got the worst hiding of my entire life. The next day I got myself to the hospital. They were shocked and they took photos of the cuts, and when the police got hold of that I never got sent back to my relatives. I was sent back to my mum. My mum! I get to see my mum. I was 11 or 12.

When I saw my mum, the state that she was in, she was a stranger to me. She had been on methamphetamine, which completely changed the way that she looked, how she acted. It wasn't the mum I had imagined. She didn't really love me.

Then I started doing weird stuff – smashing my head on brick walls, wrecking the house. I put a knife to my sister's throat, I stole alcohol to get wasted – anything to try and release whatever I was going through.

It was real dark. When I think of that house, all I see is shadows. I was like, Fuck the world; I'm going to do what I want. That was my mentality. Hope? I don't think I knew what that was. No hope at all. I had no goals, I had no dreams.

Elliot: Levi describes some horrific early life experiences. However, even less severe events like *difficulties in the home* can be a risk factor: this can include unstable caregiving or inconsistent caregiving techniques. While some children adapt smoothly to shifting demands – either from a parent who is inconsistent in their approach or across parents and homes – others struggle.

Parental conflict and *illness in the family* can be triggers for a young person to slip, sometimes unnoticed, into depression. When their parents are arguing, many young people feel that it's somehow their fault and, perhaps obviously, their sense of security is undermined.

When the attention is all towards an ill family member, the young person might feel jealous, angry or sad. We see this in Alex's story.

Alex (Hannah's sister): Hannah was the main priority at home, and there was a lot of arguing. I would get pissed off with Mum and Dad. It felt like they were favouring Hannah: she was getting all the attention. It would make me feel hate towards Hannah. I'd come home and there'd be no one home and there'd be a note saying, 'We're at the hospital with Hannah.' It was hard to come home to just that. Normally I'd come home and call out 'Hi'. For me it was like, Hannah's getting all this attention, and they're always together and that's who they care about. Now I understand it was because of Hannah's health.

Elliot: Ralph Waldo Emerson, the nineteenth-century essayist and poet, said that temperament 'is the iron wire on which the beads [of life] are strung'. Temperament is what is generally referred to as the biological component of someone's personality (as opposed to the learnt component, or character).

Temperament can be a risk factor. If your child is less adaptable by disposition, they may recover less easily from the sadnesses that affect us all, and be more susceptible to developing depression. However, other temperaments can be protective: a child who is by nature social and who can adjust easily to change and to different situations is less likely to develop depression.

When parents separate, or a parent dies, a young person will experience *grief and loss*. These are really normal feelings. But some young people will get stuck in a cycle of unhappiness and perhaps even self-blame.

Other kinds of loss can also play a role – relationship break-ups, loss of a grandparent or friend, loss of self-esteem through trouble with the law, perceived family disappointment or bullying.

When there are a number of these stressors building on each other, the person's vulnerability really increases.

Bullying and *unpopularity or isolation* are other risk factors. It is a terrible thing for a teenager to feel that they don't fit in, and even worse if they are bullied. If your child is lonely and has not settled into a comfortable peer group, they are at higher risk of depression than a child who is socially settled. Hayley's story is a poignant reminder of this.

Given that *identity formation* is such a huge part of adolescence, it's no surprise that challenges in this area can make someone more vulnerable. Questions for someone around their gender identity and sexual orientation can be particularly confusing and challenging for a young person, particularly if accompanied with isolation or bullying from others.

A confident sense of *belonging and cultural identity* are significant protective factors for young people. Their absence, however, can be another area of potential vulnerability, for instance for Maori young people with no connection to their iwi or hapu.

Young Maori suffer disproportionately from mental illness; and young Maori males have the greatest burden of all. The New Zealand Mental Health Survey found that mental disorder was higher for Maori and Pacific people than for anyone else; and that in the past 12 months the prevalences were 29.5% for Maori, 24.4% for Pacific people and 19.3% for Others, which indicates that Maori and Pacific people have a greater burden due to mental health problems. Much of this burden appears to be because of the youthfulness of the Maori and Pacific populations and their relative socio-economic disadvantage. Young Pacific people born in New Zealand to Pacific Island-born parents have the added stress of living with their family's cultural expectations and also living within the different values of New Zealand culture.

Amitai: I was raised by parents who'd come over to New Zealand from Samoa and just knuckled down. They experienced hardships and they got through them. Handle it – that's their approach to life; and I feel like they projected that on to us: We've done it; you push through.

My parents were very critical of the things I would do, especially my public speaking. My grandfather was a great orator, so I was expected to be the same. Sometimes when I would become anxious and upset about their harsh feedback, they would say 'What are you crying for?' I knew that showing emotion was not a good thing, so I learnt to bottle things up.

- If a child has an episode of depression before they turn 18, they have an increased chance of another episode before they turn twenty-four.
- Stressful life events can trigger mental disorders, increase risk for depression, trigger depression and sometimes contribute to keeping it going (see box below).
- Young people sometimes blame themselves for the things that happen in their families.
- Identity and belonging are crucial for wellbeing, and a lack of these can increase vulnerability.
- Young Maori suffer disproportionately in mental illness, and young Maori males have the greatest burden of all.
- Young Pacific people have the added stress of living with their family's cultural expectations, within the different values of New Zealand culture.

Key risk factors for mental illness

- genetics
- temperament/personality style
- parental modelling or coping
- stressful events
- abuse (sexual, physical, emotional)
- family difficulties – inconsistent parenting, parental conflict
- loss – of a parent, significant person, key relationship, self-esteem
- bullying or social isolation
- identity formation issues
- confused sense of belonging, lack of or conflicted cultural identity

PART THREE

Getting Help

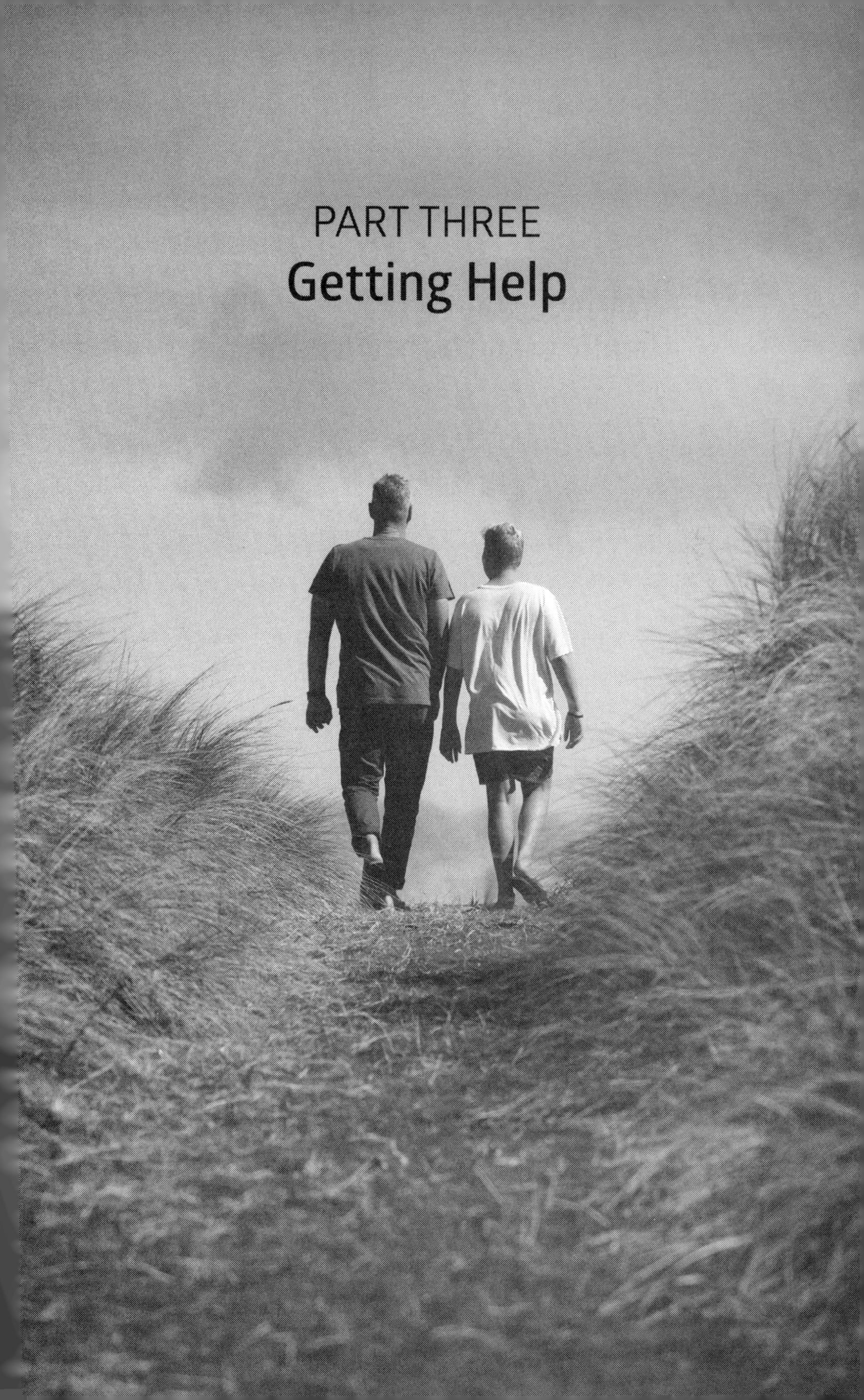

16.
'Nothing should resonate more loudly than your own intuition'

Catherine (Sean's mum): My husband and I had been away for the weekend to celebrate my fiftieth birthday, and when we arrived home Sean, who was 15, met us at the door in floods of tears. He kept saying, 'I don't know why I feel like this, because if you look at everything in my life I have the perfect life.' I thought, *Sean, you are depressed. It's not your fault. It's nothing to be ashamed of and we need help for you.*

My immediate response was to phone a counsellor. She didn't get back to me straight away, and by the time she did Sean had decided he wasn't going to see anybody. Even though he did appear to improve after that big cry and a couple of days off school, I wonder, in retrospect, whether taking what he said at face value and not insisting that he saw the counsellor was a mistake on my part. That gives me some feelings of guilt. I read a very good line recently: 'Nothing should resonate more loudly than your own intuition', and it's certainly true when you're dealing with your own child. I probably didn't follow my own intuition at that point. That gives me some feeling of guilt even now.

JK: When it comes to my kids, I am wary about medicalising them too soon. I am interested in being aware of their character, and parenting in a way that acknowledges who they are and what their needs are. That's the first thing to think of.

Does anxiety turn into depression? It can make someone more vulnerable to it, for sure. OK, can I deal with my child's anxiety? Can I find out what he's really anxious about? Can I find out more about how I can parent it? For me, in the normal course of life, that's not a call for an early diagnosis: that's understanding the character of your child.

I want to understand how different characteristics can act together in the personality of a child. Like in my own case, for example: was it shyness, together with poor self-esteem, together with insecurity that contributed to me getting depressed? How could those character traits have been parented so as not to contribute to depression? I want to recognise the early signs so it doesn't become an illness and we don't need to 'diagnose' it.

If I saw some of those characteristics in my child I might go, OK, he's got some anxiety issues that I need to address. And *I'd* get the help before I got *him* the help. I'd say, How can I parent this? I would talk to him, try and get him to understand his fears, try and give him some strategies to feel more in control. That's how I'd try to parent for resilience.

But I keep coming back to the fact that it's an illness. You can do all the screening you want, but bad stuff can still happen. Yes, we want to break down the stigma, give people educational tools and parenting tools where we can create resilience – but the kid might still have anxiety or depression. Some people will always fall through the net, like I did myself.

With our kids, we do everything we can, but they still might get sick. *It's an illness.* And if you get onto it early, your chances of recovery are really good. So: let's create resilience in our kids. But if someone does become unwell then it's no big deal – we see the doctor, we see the psychologist, we create a team to work together on the problem, we keep parenting for resilience, we even encourage our young people to take the pills if necessary. That's the way I look at it.

There's no shame in it. This is what we do with physical complaints. If your son has a rash you think about what's causing it and you try to treat it yourself, and if it doesn't go away you go to the doctor for their expertise and input.

Kirsty: As a parent or caregiver of a young person it's not your job to diagnose depression or anxiety disorders. However, you are in a unique position to spot some of the warning signs, assist the young person to access support and walk alongside them, supporting them on their recovery journey.

We would really like to acknowledge how challenging this is. It is inevitable that you will question yourself: How bad does it have to be before I should take action or seek professional help? Am I overreacting?

Keep an eye out for some of the warning signs we've noted (see chapter 12). Be aware if your young person has a number of the risk factors. We would say, if you're not sure but you have a gut feeling that things are not quite right, the earlier you can get some input and some support, the better. The longer it is left, the more challenging it can become for the teen to engage in strategies to help themselves. Strain can also develop in relationships as the illness impacts on the teen's ability to engage with you: there is a good chance it will be really stressful for you. Schooling and developmental tasks can be disrupted, and secondary issues such as self-medication with alcohol and drugs can develop.

There is no harm in seeking support and having these conversations early. In fact they can be preventive. Even if a health professional tells you that it isn't 'bad/serious/severe enough' for them to have ongoing input, a one-off session can still be useful to tell you and the teen what to watch out for and how to manage any current concerns and build on strengths.

Things can change pretty quickly for adolescents – like they did for Sean. They can say things are really bad, and then one of the stressors shifts, such as a relationship, and they feel better. Whether the shift is temporary or more permanent, I think these are still great windows of opportunity. It's an opportunity to acknowledge the hard stuff, promote help-seeking, identify some strategies and show your support: 'I'm really glad things are feeling a bit better for you now; I was really worried about you.' 'You probably don't feel you need them right now, but let's use this as an opportunity to find out some options in case things do get pretty bad again.' 'It's sometimes hard to find strategies/supports when things aren't going well, so let's find out about some now that you could maybe call on next time you're feeling low or something really bad happens.'

Elliot: Depression and anxiety are serious illnesses that cause a lot of distress, but they are both treatable, and the sooner you seek diagnosis and treatment for your young person, the better. As we've noted, if left untreated they can have really serious consequences for ongoing quality of life – even on the ability to just function in life. So if your young person has some of the risk factors and you've seen some of the warning signs, trust your instincts: talk to them and assist them to get the support they need.

- If you're worried, the earlier you get some input and some support, the better.
- There is no harm in seeking support and having these conversations early. In fact, they can be preventive.
- Untreated, depression and anxiety can have really serious consequences for a teen's ability to function and for their ongoing quality of life.

17. Labelling – now I know why I feel this way

Elliot: One of the difficulties with depression is that it can look like something else. It can look like 'bad' behaviour. Or it can seem like depression but actually be a thyroid problem, or some other illness; or maybe it is depression but the depression is a response to some other physical or psychiatric condition. So it's a good idea for a GP to be your first port of call. Clinical diagnosis of a young person's anxiety or depression is a really important start.

But as soon as you get into this territory of 'diagnosis' people start worrying about 'labelling'. *I don't want my child to have a label.* You wonder: *will I have to tick the box on certain forms – say on a school application, where they ask if your child has had a mental health diagnosis? Or if they travel, will they have to tick a box saying they've had mental health services involvement in the past year?*

People can feel stigmatised, and not want the label. They can feel like they're being put in a box that will lead others to limit them or make assumptions about the person that they are – a box that suddenly defines them. They might even put themselves in that box. When you think about the spectrum that a label can traverse between 'you're depressed' or 'you're not depressed', it's also concerning – there's a lot that a mere label doesn't tell us.

However, a diagnosis or 'label' can be helpful, too – although, of course, it depends on how it's going to be used. One of the incredibly useful things about a diagnosis is that it normalises people's experience. *Oh, this is what the problem is.* You can find out more about it, and you can access a full range of support groups and information about people who are going through similar experiences – or other parents who are going through similar things with their young people. So there's an immediate sense of interconnectedness and not being alone or isolated. *There are millions of people out there experiencing something like what I'm going through. Anxiety and depression are part of the human experience and I'm not alone in this.* You can say to yourself: *now I've got a name for it; I know what it is.* You realise: *this hopelessness and this dislike for myself, that's part of this illness.* That knowledge is very empowering and can be a real relief.

Mel (Hannah's mum): A formal diagnosis immediately gives you access to resources – to helpful medication, and to a set of strategies that can be put in place.

Kirsty: As Mel notes, a label or diagnosis can also open up a wealth of resources and information for both you and your young person – information about what is going on, about what other people have found helpful, and about what works according to the research. Information about how to get through.

Getting a diagnosis can also allow the person to separate themselves from the illness: *It's an illness; it's not you, it's not who you are.* The diagnosis is of the illness, not of the person. That's one of the first things I do when I'm working with a family, with a young person, even with adult clients – I talk about it, externalise it as 'the depression' or 'the anxiety'. We talk about the depression's impact on them, so they're separate from it. Naming it puts it in its place as something that the parent and the teen (and others such as health professionals, school and family) can team up and work with. The fight is now not between the parent and the teen; now it's parent and teen working together to put the anxiety or depression in its place. The parent is standing by the young person, rather than against them. You can talk in terms of recognising when the anxiety or depression is being the boss, and together you can figure out how to 'boss back' or, as JK says, turn around and embrace it and take away some of its power. In that sense, the diagnosis can be very much a tool for recovery.

Sometimes adolescents come up with a name for it: they might call it something else, like the black cloud, the blues, the worries. Naming it externalises it, and can be an immensely useful first step. There's a fantastic book by Matthew Johnstone, *I Had a Black Dog,* that does this in a really powerful way.

So the usefulness of a diagnosis or label can come down to our and others' understanding of what that label means, the stigma that gets attached to it, and then how it's used by ourselves and others.

- People worry that a diagnosis will lead to labelling and stigma.
- Labelling is of the illness, not the person.
- The positive thing about a label is that it normalises people's experience, and enables access to information and support.
- Getting a diagnosis can allow the young person to separate themselves from the illness, and allows the parent and young person to team up together to manage it.

18.
Stigma – there are people out there who just don't get it

JK: The stigma is what stops people seeking help. It makes people blame themselves for being ill. But if you get the flu, is it your fault? If you get cancer, is it your fault? Mental illness can happen to anyone – it is unprejudiced.

When I was ill I wanted to keep it quiet because of the stigma. I was afraid. I didn't understand it as an illness, and I didn't want to be perceived as a failure or as weak. Then my psychiatrist said to me: 'If you were playing rugby and you tore a hamstring, would that be a weakness?'

'No,' I said, 'I just got injured and I need to get better.'

Now I know that depression is the same – it's just something that happens that you need to get help with, to get on the wellness track. No judgment.

My work for more than 10 years now has been about helping people understand this illness so that we can continue to break down the stigma.

Starting out, I had a lot of fear about exposing myself, but it's turned into an incredibly humbling and satisfying journey.

Jacob: It's so unbelievable to think that there are people out there who don't understand. My dad's one of them, and his mates. I was telling one of his friends about this book, and they were like, 'Oh, what a whole lot of shit. What's JK got to be unhappy about? We're all unhappy – just move on' – that kind of attitude. There are people out there who just don't get it. I think I was very influenced by that kind of attitude in my feelings toward myself.

With my depression, I blamed myself for what I was putting others through. I felt very guilty. I hated myself. A lot of self-prejudice. That general view came from Dad and elsewhere. It's our culture, partly.

You can say you've got a physical illness, but you can't say you've got depression.

Layla (Christie's mum): The campaigns have helped, but we've still got a long way to go. When it happens to us, we mustn't feel that we're weak or to blame. You never know what might be round the corner for you, and it's really important not to judge and not to blame.

Sophie: There's a stigma to do with depression. It's like a title you're given. It's hard to tell other people you're going through it. People think that depression is something you can control. It's like, 'Snap out of it.'

Scarlet: With teens it might still be a bit embarrassing to admit it because you're not sure how people might respond. They might act a bit weird around you if they know you've got this condition. So I guess there is a fear of how people will react.

Kirsty: One of the big issues around diagnosis and labelling is this matter of stigma. We have come a long way in destigmatising mental illness, but nevertheless there is a lot of fear and, as Layla said, we still have a way to go.

I wonder if part of the stigma attached to mental illness is that people seldom talk about it in its mild to moderate stages. They manage it internally as a family, either on their own or with professional help, but they don't talk about it publicly. So the 'public view' of depression is often when it's at the more severe end and the young person has turned to alcohol and drugs, which kids typically do to self-manage their emotions; or when bad behaviour gets them kicked out of school; or when they make a suicide attempt. Those behaviours are more extreme, and other people, when their own kid starts to experience mental health issues, can't relate to that extreme picture. They don't understand that it's one part of the spectrum that might occur, but doesn't always.

I think we've created our own vicious circle: we're not allowing the full range of mental illness to be talked about or acknowledged, so people's picture of it in their heads is something that they can't relate to.

Of course, it's the extremes that tend to get media coverage, too. People see a news items about an extreme rare behaviour that gets tagged to someone's mental illness, and without the full knowledge of what depression, anxiety or psychosis are, they panic and think: *My child doesn't have that*.

A related issue is that, because of stigma and fear, people don't look for help until they're at the extreme end. There is a lot of information about prevention, about how to intervene early, but people don't pick up the books or visit the website until the symptoms have really taken hold. Remember: the earlier you see the signs, the earlier you identify the problem, the better chance you have of managing it and lessening its negative impact.

Amitai: I definitely think in our Pacific communities there is a lot of stigma around the unseen illness. If it's something to do with depression especially, it's kind of like: 'Mate, get over it. Harden up.'

It's an attitude that I took on when I was younger. When you experience something that's difficult emotionally, or you're mentally overwhelmed, you feel like you're weak; you're just not strong enough to do what's being asked of you, even though there's no physical strength required. In my experience it's been hard for many Pacific people to accept and comprehend mental distress or illness without associating it with an unacceptable form of weakness. It's like double standards: it's not your fault if you have cancer; if you break your leg you'll receive support, understanding and time to recover. But if you experience depression, you're just expected to suck it up and carry on because it's not a real illness.

You start to scold yourself because it's like you can't handle 'normal' things in life and you don't know why. You begin to feel incompetent and frustrated. And you hear these voices in your head that you shouldn't be like this.

My parents always used to say, 'You don't have an excuse to be like that.' I thought from an early age that experiencing mental illness or depression wasn't a real thing, so I would feel stupid if I asked for help.

Kirsty: The reality is that stigma about anything can take generations to overcome. So, while there's a lot more public awareness now about mental illness – some great TV ads, books and websites – there are still plenty of people around us who were brought up in a different way, with certain beliefs and prejudices. And often those people – the parents, the grandparents – still govern family attitudes: 'Oh, there's nothing wrong with them. A bunch of whingers. They don't know how lucky they've got it. They should just snap out of it . . .'

I think it will be something that shifts as the generations go by, and chipping away at it is very important. There are so many positive signs. Schools are becoming more literate in mental health. Youth workers and health professionals are much better informed; and there's a huge growth in online support and resources. Perhaps most importantly, role models in sports, music and business as well as 'everyday people' are putting their hands up and saying, 'Mental illness is a part of my life and I'm OK. It's not because I'm weak or different or not capable – it's just an illness.'

The Mental Health Foundation recently ran a competition in schools for kids to design a video to make people stop and think when they hear cruel and hurtful words like 'nutjob', 'retard', 'schizo' or 'mental', and reflect on language that is stigmatising or discriminatory. Things like this both reflect and encourage a real shift in attitudes and a hope that, in future, there will be less stigma towards those suffering any kind of mental illness.

Now we need to focus on families. A part of destigmatising mental illness depends on families being comfortable talking about it. We know that parents often feel uncomfortable talking about mental health and mental illness with their children, or sharing their own experiences with mental illness. Sometimes this is because of the stigma, or anxiety about whether it will change their child's view of them. It may be because the adult is not happy with the way their experience of mental illness was managed, and doesn't want to share that with the child. There may be a sense of hopelessness and 'predestination' as they encounter some of the same symptoms in their child.

However, things are different now: their teen may have a different temperament, different experiences, different environment, different resources, different professional knowledge, and different parental knowledge. Because of their own experience, the adult can help them identify it earlier and get the support they need.

If this is the case for you, talking with your young person about your own mental illness experiences doesn't have to be a big, intense conversation. By referring to it like you might refer to other experiences you had growing up, you immediately destigmatise it: *this is part of who I am*. You can refer to things you've seen in the paper or on TV or in a conversation: 'You know, I experienced something like that when I was growing up' or 'I don't know if Dad's mentioned it to you, but I was pretty anxious when I was younger' or 'I had periods of being really low when I was in my teens.' Acknowledge the hard parts of it, but also emphasise that you came through; or that it's just part of your life and that you continue to function normally with it. Above all, let them know they can talk to you about it at any stage if they want, and if they have any concerns. If it's something you're still struggling with, you can emphasise how you wish you had got more support when you were younger, and talk about taking the wellness journey together.

Mental illness is so common, and yet because of the stigma we all struggle along on our own, not feeling we can talk about it or share the load. This only increases the stress.

Breaking down stigma has to occur on multiple levels. We have to keep speaking out, saying that mental illness is not a weakness, it's an illness and lots of people have it, it looks like this, there are treatments, and people can live very whole lives. It is not a skeleton in the closet! It's all of our responsibility to do this.

A journey to self-acceptance

Amitai: Self-acceptance is a crucial part of my mental health. It's something I'm much better at now but am still working on.

I work in a largely Pacific organisation and I wouldn't tell them two things: I wouldn't tell them I'm gay; and I wouldn't tell them I've had an experience of depression. So there's still a long way to go in terms of learning how to cope with the stigma within our culture towards both of those things. As a man who thinks he's pretty resilient and good at persevering, it's still hard for me to accept that, yes, I experienced a time of mental distress and suicidal ideation, a time where I needed help and couldn't cope, because we're indoctrinated to think it's a sign of weakness.

But now that I am an adult I can challenge some of those ideas, both in myself and in the culture around me. It's only now as an adult that I can say, 'That's not the way we should be responding to things.' Often as young people we don't have that ability to go, 'Don't say that to me.' We're not reassured that it's natural not to be mentally healthy all the time, and that there are actually ways we can manage our mental wellbeing better, rather than just ignoring it and hoping the situation changes.

Having said that, I'm optimistic because, in terms of PI cultural views, I know we have a culture of love and service when we understand and embrace the uniqueness of everyone's situation. Pacific people often go beyond the call of duty when serving their families and communities. They have some of the biggest hearts, so I know there is great potential for us to do better.

There is a long road ahead. In my adulthood I choose not to believe that the conditions perpetuating my distress around accepting my sexuality were symptomatic of 'Pacific values'. I give my community more credit than that. However, when I was younger it was much harder not to believe that my family, church and community hated a part of me that I couldn't change.

Pacific cultures are not filled with hate and fear; they are centred on the connection of all things. We understand the importance of the 'sacred spaces between' which must be 'made beautiful' in our interactions with one another. So there is a lot of work to be done to make sure young people can genuinely feel and experience this connectedness and feel safe to navigate their own journeys forward.

In the organisation that I work for, I know enough now to realise that some of my colleagues will have experienced depression or anxiety, but nobody talks about it. Maybe that's a challenge for the future.

Stigma – there are people out there who just don't get it

- Although public education campaigns have helped a lot, there is still stigma surrounding mental illness.
- Because of stigma and fear, people often don't look for help until they're at the more severe end of mental illness.
- We all play a role in reducing stigma, and an important step will be when families are comfortable talking about mental illness.
- If you have experienced mental illness, sharing this with your teen in a constructive way can be very helpful.

19.
Teamwork

JK: Depression is the modern illness and I believe it comes out of, or at least is made worse by, the dominant kind of lifestyle and culture that we have. Stress and depression – when you're in that situation, the only way to deal with it is through teamwork.

The team we create around ourselves to help us through dark times is not that different to a sports team. When I'm putting a sports team together, I make sure I've created a whole. So, since I'm a big-picture person, I need to find detail people. I call it the pizza – my skills make up this segment, and my other coaches come in and deliver their expertise, and that makes up the whole pizza. Together, we create a whole. And that's what makes a team – any kind of team: different skills, different strengths, all pulling together for a common goal. We all have our own responsibilities, and where the crossover is, that's where we get connectivity – I need to connect with these guys and they need to connect with me.

When it comes to mental health and making a team that's going to work for you when someone in the family's unwell or struggling, it's no different. It's about strengths and weaknesses. You might have the EQ – the emotional intelligence – that is your love for your child and your understanding, your gut instinct, that they're not well. But you need the IQ – the actual knowledge and understanding of skilled people who can help you and tell you what to do. *Give us the IQ around our EQ.* That's what we want from all the professionals.

The importance of teamwork in anything is fundamental. Teamwork is about knowing you can't do it all yourself.

Family is hugely important to my players. I say to them, you can't say to me that you're playing for your family and then not go out and give it all on the football field. I'm talking about commitment. We're committed to our families. We'll do anything. We'll go the extra mile every time. So let's go the extra mile and put a good team together to look after our kids.

Elliot: I want to emphasise the importance of families and their role in helping a young person recover from mental illness. My own philosophy of care is this: that the most powerful combination of inputs is a young person, the professional people and the family, all on the same page and all working together. If you can achieve that, you have something that is very powerful.

Parents have such an intimate knowledge of their kids. It astounds me when mental health professionals don't seek collateral information from the people who know their clients well. It's almost the first thing I'm thinking about: Who are their family? Who are the key people in this person's life? Of course, it's not always straightforward, and there can be tangled family dynamics, but in general the family is crucial in the process.

I do want to acknowledge how incredibly stressful this is for parents. Not only do you have your concerns about your child, and possibly your frustration and grief at the way they are changing, but you might be becoming aware of your lack of knowledge about services. Perhaps you have a partner who sees things differently (perhaps you're worrying but they're saying, 'She'll be right, stop fussing'). And perhaps your young person is denying there's a problem and saying they don't want to go to the doctor. You might be feeling all sorts of challenging feelings: guilt that somehow you caused this problem; anger at your young person for not snapping out of it or being grateful for what they have; hopelessness around what to do; fear about what is happening to your child and what the future might hold; sadness at the loss of your old relationship with your child. These feelings are difficult to deal with and at times immensely overwhelming and paralysing – but they're absolutely normal.

We suggest beginning by finding someone you can talk to about all this, who you can trust to be supportive and understanding. This may be your partner, or it may be a friend or relative who has some experience of mental illness, or it may be a good friend you know you can lean on. This person will be an important member of your personal team.

It's likely that the first professional person you need to get on your team is your GP. GPs can facilitate entry to the mental health services. Most are experienced and sensitive about the mental health needs of their patients – it's a big part of their work. You should expect to feel heard and to have a sense of moving forward after a consultation with them. If not, you're perfectly within your rights to find another GP for a second opinion.

Most people will probably go to their regular family doctor, and in most cases that is the best starting point. Your GP will be able to do an assessment, and can either refer you directly on to a mental health clinic for further assessment, or make a recommendation regarding other types of support options that might be available to you.

The family GP may not always be the right choice for an adolescent, perhaps because adolescent mental health might not be an area of their expertise, or perhaps because your young person might not feel comfortable discussing their issues with someone they see as having a strong alliance with their parents and family. On the other hand, your young person might feel safer talking to a GP whom they have known for a long time.

In the bigger centres you could ask whether there are doctors in the practice who specialise in mental health issues, or who are particularly comfortable working with adolescents. There may be a Youth One Stop Shop, which is a youth-focused community-based health centre that often has specific youth GP services. In rural communities this is more difficult, and you may need to ask around and perhaps even travel to the next town. We highly recommend the Youth One Stop Shops, but they are available only in a few centres.

Mel (Hannah's mum): At one point, my feelings of fear and inadequacy mobilised me to make a list and get in touch with the 14 people I'd identified as being our 'team' – from the GP to the social worker, the psychiatrist to the head nurse at the paediatric ward. I sent them an email saying, 'I have recognised that those listed above are our team and at this point I don't know if any one of you is leading this team. I would like you to come back to me and tell me who is leading this team, on the basis that if the worst is to happen, and it feels like it might at the moment, where does the buck stop? I'm not looking for blame but for leadership.'

I think it's really good, if you've done your own research, to be able to say to your GP or whatever person you're seeing, 'I've heard *this*' – and print it out and have it with you. 'What do you think about this? I appreciate you might not have seen it yet, would you be interested in seeing it?' I think the willingness of the clinician to say, 'Thanks, please send me more,' is very telling. My favourite doctor is like that, and sure enough was an important member of my team.

I would recommend looking for a health provider who empowers the parent or whoever to do the job. It's about a team: health professionals recognising the importance of that family and friend role, and supporting them.

- Teamwork is an essential part of dealing with mental illness.
- Families have a vital role in helping a young person recover from mental illness. The most powerful combination of inputs is a young person, the professional people and the family, all on the same page and all working together.
- Build your own team, starting with someone you trust to be supportive and understanding. Then add professionals such as doctors, mental health services, and so on.
- Be sensitive about your choice of doctor – your family GP may or may not be the best choice for your teenager.

20.
The first step of a long journey

JK: Getting a diagnosis is important, but it's only the first step. Sometimes the scariest moments are after you've been diagnosed. You'd think that by opening up and talking about it, it's going to go away – but it doesn't. You're not going to wake up tomorrow and be fine. It's like, just knowing you've got a broken bone doesn't mend it, does it? And it's the same for depression and anxiety and related disorders. Getting a diagnosis is the first step of a long journey. You've got to get treatment and then you've got to wait and see.

The biggest shift for me was when I accepted the illness for what it was, and then worked on it. I reached out for help, and that was the first step towards my recovery.

Marie: At the age of 15, our daughter Isabella started having panic attacks at school, and they became more frequent and spiralled quickly into self-harm and depression.

Isabella was the child we never worried about – she was so laidback, always so happy and cheerful – so it really can happen to anyone. She became hypersensitive to stuff that she'd never been sensitive about before. She became really anxious about homework. It was a definite change from before. That very quickly developed into panic attacks at school – literally these collapses, meltdowns; she couldn't breathe – physical, horrible things that got her down so badly.

She was very quickly depressed and didn't want to go to school. She began self-harming and cutting herself. She said it made her feel better. She said it was a real relief. And she admitted she was also purging, throwing up after eating. We wouldn't have thought to ask, but she told us because she wanted help, in a moment of clarity. I saw the purging as another form of self-harm – having a go at herself, trying to sort out her emotions. She also got really drunk all by herself.

Because another family member had previously been ill with an anxiety disorder we were able to very quickly recognise what was going on with Isabella, and we swung into action immediately. We took her to the GP, who referred us to the local adolescent mental health service. She began taking antidepressants, as well as beginning with a therapist. The antidepressants took a long time to have an effect, and in the end a psychiatrist prescribed her a different one, which made sense as it was one that had worked well for other family members.

We didn't force her to go to school: there was no battle around any of that. And we said to Isabella: 'We've got you, darling. We know what's happening. This is bloody awful but you're going to be OK. We're going to get you through this and we're going to help you do it. We're taking control. I know you think I'm smothering you but I'm not – I'm here because I care, and when I know that you're better, that you're well enough, I'll be able to let you go.'

We didn't say, 'Tell us how you are feeling . . . How? . . . Why?'

We knew she needed to be kept safe. We told her, 'You're safe with us.' Mostly she just accepted it; and I wouldn't hesitate to do it again. This was a strong lesson we'd learned from my sister's experience with her daughter.

Isabella is nearly 16 now. She's still on medication – and will be for another six months because I want to well and truly get her better – but she's going to school every day happily, living a normal life.

Elliot: As we can see from Isabella's story, medication can have its place. Furthermore a combination of medicine and therapy – in particular, cognitive behaviour therapy (CBT) – can be highly effective in treating anxiety and depression, especially when treatment begins early. Medication alleviates symptoms, and therapy improves a person's self-knowledge and their ability to self-monitor and self-care, and greatly reduces the risk of further episodes of serious depression or anxiety.

With treatment, 70–80 percent of people with depression will recover more quickly, and for most there will be a complete recovery, according to our own Ministry of Health figures. Those findings are echoed in many international studies.

But even if you're doing everything right, it can be a long journey. And it's a hard one, too, as JK points out. It can feel quite overwhelming at times. However, it's important not to interpret that overwhelmingness as meaning you're not on the right track or that it won't get better. Instead, we need to acknowledge that it's normal and understandable to sometimes feel overwhelmed because it is a difficult process. Not only is the mental health system reasonably complex, but the natural pathways that mental health recovery takes can be very complex and challenging. There are few straight lines in mental health recovery.

JK: I saw this great drawing about recovery the other day that shows exactly what Elliot is saying. It's definitely something I can relate to!

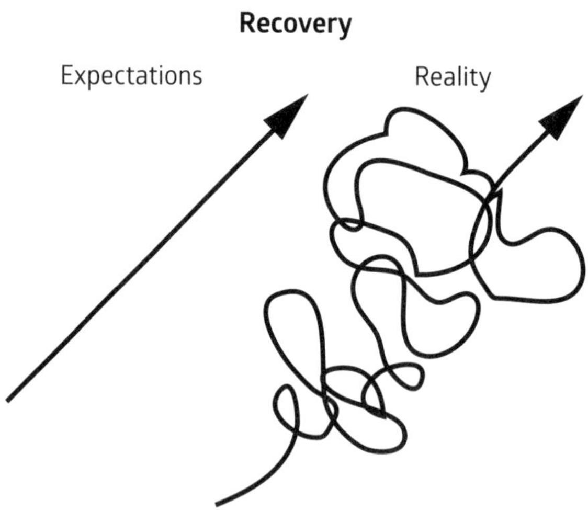

Elliot: Without treatment, an episode of depression may last six to nine months or more, with a high chance of recurrence. Some people with depression will not get better on their own.

And if the strategies haven't been learned to manage it the first time around, the person is at much greater risk the second time around. This is because the levels of hopelessness can be much higher: *I thought I was over it, but here I am again. Oh, man, I can't have another six months of this . . .* versus: *I know this, I recognise it for what it is. I've beaten it once before: I know what I need to put in place.*

Being able to put strategies in place increases psychological wellbeing, in part because of the great benefits of taking charge and feeling more in control.

Sometimes young people can be diagnosed with mild to moderate depression and they go on medication and very soon the symptoms begin to lift – and maybe something good happens, like a new relationship – and they think, *oh, I don't really need the therapy or to talk with anyone about what went on.*

I think that's a shame and a missed opportunity, because the education base of therapy is immensely helpful – both the education about what depression or anxiety is, and also what it looks like for this person: What are their warning signs? What are their triggers? and, obviously, What would they do if they started to feel like that again? It can really help, in the future, if things don't go well again and the depression reoccurs. You can learn what you need to put in place. It's a support that you can come back to.

- You have to be very patient. Getting a diagnosis is the first step of what can be a long process. The earlier this process and treatment begin, the better.
- The case for therapy is clear; and there can also be a place for medication. Furthermore, a combination of medicine and therapy can be highly effective.
- Therapy improves a person's self-knowledge and greatly reduces the risk of further episodes of serious depression.
- It's normal and understandable to sometimes feel overwhelmed, because it is a difficult process. There are few straight lines in recovery.

21.
Getting to the doctor

Mel (Hannah's mum): I don't think mental illness is taught well to GPs. My experience with a range of GPs leads me to ask: How can they be jacks of all trades? Some are great, some are not.

JK: You go to a concert to hear a great singer; you watch a movie for the great acting. If you're not well you go to the doctor.

There's absolutely no fear in going and talking to the doctor about not being well. It's what they're there for. They're not going to judge you. They see 50 people a day with all sorts of weird and wonderful things. There's not a lot that your GP hasn't heard, seen or looked at.

If you're worried about what people will think, well, lie! I give you full permission to lie. 'Why are you going to the doctor?' 'I've got the flu; I've had a sore throat for a month.' I'll forgive you. Depression will forgive you. Later, when and if the time is right, you can tell people what was going on; but to begin with, the important thing is to get well.

If your kid doesn't want to go to the doctor, have a look into their worries. Maybe they're thinking, *I might meet someone in the reception area that I know*; or *someone from school might see me going*; or *he might not understand me*. Answer some of the questions: 'You're not going because you need him to understand you. You're going because you need some information.'

Kirsty: JK is right – it can sometimes be difficult getting a young person to seek help. Keep in mind how long it may have taken you to work up to feeling comfortable with the idea. If it took you a while, it may take them a while, too; you can't expect them to embrace the idea immediately. In the meantime, you could go to your GP or have a consult with some services yourself, as a starting point. This could be very useful for building your confidence, and it might also give you more concrete things to say to your teen about the process, and about what exactly would happen during a visit to the doctor.

Remember they may be feeling stigma and not wanting to draw attention to themselves. Also, the symptoms of depression – hopelessness, lack of motivation and energy – will also be working against them wanting to seek help.

We suggest having a conversation where you don't complain about their behaviour or judge them, just highlight your concerns. This can be really hard. One way of taking the judgment out of a conversation is to simply describe to them what you see: 'I'm worried about some of the changes in your behaviour. You stayed in bed all weekend; you're unable to get up to go to school; you didn't eat your dinner last night; and you've stopped going out with your friends. I'm also really concerned about the things you are saying, such as that everything is pointless.'

Reassure them that you love them, and that you are looking out for them.

The psychiatrist Lloyd Sederer has a good suggestion: 'You can also try saying: Often there are two different parts in all of us – the part that wants to stay the same and the part that wants to change. I am on the side that wants to change and get better. What I take from all the ways you are behaving, whether you say so or not, is that you are calling out for help.'

Emphasise that mental illnesses such as depression and anxiety are real, and that they affect how a person thinks, acts and feels – including their motivation to get help. Try and keep externalising the problem, rather than making them the problem. Compare what they're experiencing to a physical illness or injury – for instance, a chest infection or a stretched muscle in a leg – and point out that you would go to the doctor for those things. Say things like: 'I'm not sure what's going on for you. Maybe you're not sure what's going on for you. But I'm worried about you and I want to help you to access the support you need. What I do know is that when people have hard stuff going on the earlier they get support the better they do.'

Talk openly about what they can expect, and stress that it's a confidential process – no one outside the family need know about it.

It's really important to be empathetic. Let them express concerns, and listen closely to what they say. Use these as opportunities to talk further. Encourage them to look online – for instance, thelowdown (thelowdown.co.nz) and The Journal (depression.org.nz) will have questionnaires that may give them insight and help normalise their experience and encourage them to seek help.

Emphasise that you are in this together, and that your job is to support and assist them to get better.

This can be particularly challenging if you already have difficulties in your relationship with your teen, and especially if their illness is making them more unwilling to engage – if they are irritable, withdrawn, hopeless, and so on. If this is the case you need to acknowledge the difficulties and, rather than backing right off, enlist support. Is there someone else who can help, who perhaps they would feel more comfortable going with – an aunt, youth group person, school guidance counsellor, older cousin?

Remain involved, though, and make it clear you want to be involved.

Expect there to be challenges. Talk about the role that a professional can have for a young person: 'OK, you may not like *x* and *y* about them, but they have knowledge about *z* and that could be useful for you.'

If they really don't want to go to the doctor, you could agree to wait and see for a bit. This is an option so long as the symptoms aren't disabling. But I don't mean passive waiting and seeing. You might agree not to call the doctor just yet, but in the meantime you will be monitoring and checking in, keeping a record of your concerns, getting more information, putting supports in place. This is a waiting and seeing where you are still being proactive rather than avoidant.

However, remember that the best time to intervene is early. If your concerns continue, ring the doctor.

If your teen absolutely refuses to go to the doctor, the best remaining option is for you to go yourself and outline the problem. The GP might be able to suggest the next step. The point here is to get your GP on side – enlist them in your team.

Some young people will be embarrassed about the prospect of discussing personal matters in front of their parent. Offer them the choice of having you in the consultation room or not. If they don't want you in there, ask the doctor if you can come in for the last few minutes so that you can be informed and included in the plan.

Elliot: If the GP makes an assessment and decides that your child is suffering from a clinical depression or an anxiety disorder, at that point they will probably suggest expanding your team further. You may be referred to a psychiatrist for medical advice; a psychologist or other therapist for therapy. So you now have two and possibly three professional people on your team.

It's important that you remain an active member of this team – and that means becoming informed about the illness your child has been diagnosed with, options for treatment, and the right questions to ask the professionals every step along the way. It is your right to expect quality care for your child, but no one in the process is going to love this child the way that you do. You are their main support. Some parents, like Hannah's mum Mel, even see themselves as the captain of the team.

The types of services available to provide help and professional input will depend on the severity of the depression or anxiety your teen is experiencing, the area you live in, and the primary health organisation (PHO) your GP is part of. Options can include psychological therapies through the PHO, Youth One Stop Shop supports, NGO counselling, secondary mental health services, school guidance counsellors, therapies provided by mental health professionals working in private practices, and e-therapies (thelowdown.co.nz provides a good summary of all these options). Ask your GP what resources are available in your area, whether they have a cost or session limit, and what choices you might have in terms of the types of therapies available.

- Express your concerns to your young person in non-judgmental ways: simply tell them what you have observed about their behaviour and demeanour.
- Young people sometimes do not want to go to the doctor.
- Let them express their concerns, and listen closely to what they say. Talk openly about what they can expect, and stress that it's a confidential process. Be sensitive.
- Compare what they are experiencing to a physical illness or injury, and point out that you would go to the doctor for those things. Emphasise that mental illnesses such as depression and anxiety are real, and that they affect how a person thinks, acts and feels.
- If necessary visit the doctor yourself for advice.
- Find out from your GP and online what resources are available in your area.

22.
Antidepressants

JK: I hated the idea of taking pills. At that time, the idea of pills was tied up with my ideas about personal weakness. I thought I'd be letting myself down. Now I know I was wrong: there's no weakness associated with taking antidepressants, it's just part of what it takes to get over depression.

I'd have done anything to feel better. So I began taking antidepressants, and that was part of the beginning of my journey back to wellness. I tried a couple of different types before I found the one that suited me. That was another quite lengthy process – annoying, waiting for it to kick in.

I never got complete wellness out of the pills, but they alleviated the symptoms, gave me the balance to cope; then it was up to me to start working on my wellness. So, my advice: don't expect the pills to get you well. And don't come off them too early. You've got to do both. You've got to look into yourself, and keep taking the pills.

Helene: Once I started taking the antidepressants I noticed a difference quite quickly. Definitely within a couple of weeks I was more clear-headed. The thing I was most grateful for was that they seemed to help with the racing thoughts, so I began to feel calmer and I was able to sleep. For a while there, I would cry for no reason – and they helped with that, too.

I know I was nervous when I first started taking them, because I wasn't sure what to expect. I had a bit of stigma towards taking drugs for a mental problem: I guess I had the idea that you're a stronger person if you can get through it without having to do that. I was afraid that they would change my personality or deaden my emotions – turn me into some sort of zombie. But that wasn't the case at all. I was still the same person, just not so sad and panicky.

Elliot: Antidepressants work on brain function, stabilising and normalising the neurotransmitters in our brain to alleviate symptoms.

Psychological therapies are recommended as the first line of treatment for young people with depression and anxiety, and are the preferred treatment for someone with mild to moderate depression.

Sometimes, too, a young person will be put on the medication if their symptoms are so severe that they're unable to engage in any kind of therapy. Medication can provide a boost to get to a point where they can engage.

Lyndy Matthews (psychiatrist): Depression is associated with low levels of a family of chemicals called amines – the neurotransmitters that help nerve cells to stay in touch with each other. Amines – particularly dopamine and serotonin – are carried by nerve pathways into the frontal lobe; but when their levels are low, the nerve cells in the frontal lobes become starved and that gives rise to the symptoms of depression.

An analogy I sometimes use is that depression is like a tree in winter. There is dendritic dieback – fewer connections between nerve cells. The patient can't think straight, their biology is disturbed and the world becomes a very small, miserable place. What happens with antidepressants is that it's like adding fertiliser – the amount of amines increases back to normal levels, and your dendrites, or nerve endings, grow back like a lush bush in the spring, with buds and twigs, and the connections increase. I have seen this on fast-forward electron microscopy and it's absolutely extraordinary.

Good psychotherapy does the same thing.

And that is why you have to take antidepressants for six weeks before they work, because it takes a while for those connections to grow. I say to them, 'It's not like aspirin. It's not like you're going to suddenly feel great.'

Elliot: The Best Practice Guidelines for GPs around depression in people aged under 18 recommend that antidepressant treatment should not be initiated in primary care (that is, by a GP) without consulting a psychiatrist who specialises in children and adolescents. However, given how common depression is, and the relative shortage of child and adolescent psychiatrists in New Zealand, prescribing by GPs is also common. If medication is prescribed by a GP, it's important you are confident the GP understands what contributed to the young person's depression and has presented therapy options for them as well. Without therapy, the young person can miss out on becoming aware of the way their thinking and behaviour have contributed to their depression. They might not develop healthy coping strategies to prevent relapse, or the general confidence gains that they could get with a good therapist.

Kirsty: You need to be certain that you are getting enough information from your GP – if possible, in written form. It's not uncommon for clients to say after only a week, 'It's not working.' Antidepressant medication can take up to six weeks before it becomes noticeably effective. But, possibly because of distress, some clients don't get or remember that piece of information. That's why I think a prescriber should give clear written information, and convey it in a way that the parent and the young person understand. Many GPs are fantastic on this stuff, but some are not as well informed – so go to the consultation armed with a list of questions that you want answered. We suggest that you and/or your teen ask the following.

- Why are you prescribing antidepressant medication?
- Why have you chosen this one for my condition?
- What symptoms is it targeting? For example, does it mean I won't be crying so much? Will I sleep better? Will I be able to get out of bed in the morning? Will I get my appetite back?
- How long will it take to work?
- What will I notice?
- Does it have side-effects?

- How long should I take it for?
- What are the chances my medication won't work? What will we do if it doesn't work?
- What are the other support options – e.g. therapy, support groups (for young person and family)?
- When should we come back to you for a review?

If necessary ask for a longer appointment to allow time to discuss your concerns and options properly. Inform the practice nurse that you are concerned your young person may be depressed, and that you would like a longer session if possible.

Lyndy Matthews (psychiatrist): Sometimes a person can feel a bit nauseated when they first begin taking the medication, or a bit 'la-la'. These effects don't usually last longer than a few days. To say whether an antidepressant is effective for you, you need to be on a dose every single day for six weeks.

If it works, you need to take it for at least six months, and quite possibly for up to nine or even 12 months. I use cellphone batteries as an analogy. When the battery's flat, you need to recharge it. You know what happens if you recharge your cellphone for half an hour? It tells you it's full and it works for half an hour but then it quickly goes flat again. It's exactly the same for antidepressants. It's like you have to plug in and recharge overnight, and for the human body that's six to nine months. So even though you might feel pretty much back to normal by months two or three, don't stop. People go, 'But I was feeling all right.' Don't stop! It greatly increases your chance of relapse. And even when your medication stops, you have to keep looking after yourself.

JK: I did that the first time – thought I was better and stopped taking the antidepressants too soon. That was partly because I still hadn't accepted that it was OK to be on medication. I thought I could do it myself. But I quickly went back downhill: I wasn't ready. That gave me a real wake-up call, and I went back on them.

- Psychological therapies are recommended as the first line of treatment for young people with depression.
- Antidepressants can alleviate suffering, particularly when the symptoms of depression are severe.
- Antidepressants are best prescribed for more moderate to severe depression. They work best in combination with psychotherapy.
- Take a list of questions to your doctor's appointment; and make sure you get information in writing so that you can refer to it later.
- Antidepressants can take up to six weeks to make a noticeable difference.
- When the right medication is identified, the person needs to stay on it for at least six months and quite possibly up to a year or longer.

23.
Concerns about medication

Lyndy Matthews (psychiatrist): The most common fear people have about antidepressants is that they will become addicted to them. Antidepressants are not addictive. You are not going to hang out for an antidepressant. You won't take years and need patches to get off antidepressants. People also worry about withdrawal symptoms, but it's less likely with the medication most commonly prescribed for adolescents.

Another fear young people have is that it won't be 'them' – that the medicine will fundamentally alter who they are or who they become. They worry psychiatric medicine will take away their volition, their judgment and their autonomy over their thinking processes. In fact, it's the illness that does all of that; and it often strikes me that, when patients talk about these fears, they're actually talking about their lived experience of what this illness is doing to them.

When they raise these fears, I respond by talking about the effects of untreated illness on their brain, their function, their personality and their life. I point out that the *illness* is making them 'not like their usual self'.

Kirsty: Another concern that people often want to discuss is that some antidepressants can increase the risk of suicide in adolescents. In the initial studies that prompted this concern, suicide occurred for a small subset of young people; and subsequent studies have shown varied results around this. So, while there is uncertainty regarding this issue, it needs to be carefully borne in mind by teens and by their medical practitioners when monitoring treatment and side-effects of medication.

What we do know, without a doubt, is that being depressed can increase the risk of suicide. The priority, then, is getting the most effective treatment for your young person, and if their depression is severe, then antidepressants may well need to be part of that.

It really comes down to screening and monitoring, particularly in the first few months. A challenge with medication is that it can take a few weeks to work but can have some side-effects much sooner. For a young person who is feeling overwhelmed and hopeless already, these can increase their burden at a time when they had hoped things were about to get better – and this can definitely increase feelings of hopelessness. Also, sometimes a person has to try two or three different kinds of medication before they find the one that works best for them. It's really important that the GP or psychiatrist reassure the young person and their parents about this. Part of this must be a screen for suicidal thoughts, and a discussion with the young person and the family of a plan for keeping them safe if this is a concern.

So it's not: 'We're going to the doctor and you'll get on something that will make everything go away' – which is probably what everybody is hoping. To have to slow down and face the possibility that it could go on for a while is quite a hard one to grapple with.

It's important that something is put in place to help the young person and their family through this time. Psychological therapy and education and connection with others through online sources can be incredibly helpful. The young person can begin therapy, and begin learning some of the skills that will help them.

Lyndy Matthews (psychiatrist): This is how my conversation with the teen and the parents would go in regard to safety. I would discuss with them how, as a family, they are going to manage the young person's illness. I would talk to both the parents and the young person about the antidepressants – about how the medication works; that it's going to take four to six weeks to work; that it's stimulating and it can initially make you feel a bit more anxious – and if it does, I can cover this by giving them some anti-anxiety pills. I'll acknowledge that it is going to take some weeks to turn things around.

Then I'll ask: 'Do you think you can bear it in the meantime? What are we all going to do to keep you safe, to make it manageable? How are you going to let Mum and Dad know if you're not OK?' And if the young person can't say anything, I'll look at the parents for input, and then I'll check again with the young person. I'll say something like, 'It sounds like it's really hard for you – you don't feel safe.' And they might say, 'No, I don't.' And I'll go, 'OK, well it's really important to know that. So let's talk about how we are going to keep you safe.'

What's important here is that the health professional helps to carry the worry for the family.

A key task is to support the family to care for their child; to be there for advice, to respond to concerns and to regularly review how things are going – checking that the young person is turning the corner and heading for a good recovery.

My view is that antidepressants don't kill kids. People with depression kill themselves at a much higher rate than anybody else. I haven't seen anything that shows a linear relationship between the use of antidepressants and death. But these are stimulating medications, and stimulating a depressed mind without alleviating the major symptoms can definitely put people more at risk. If that keeps us health professionals more involved for that at-risk period, sweet, we'll run with it.

The range of support options can include things like asking a family member to come and stay to help; or organising respite care, either at home or somewhere else, to give everyone a break. Support can be tailored to your needs and be altered to fit over time.

Kirsty: It is essential that there are clear expectations around what the young person and the family are to look out for, what they are to do if they are concerned at all, and when they are to come back to be checked by their GP. Just picking up the prescription from the chemist should not be an option. If your young person is taking antidepressants it is vital that they are regularly checked by their doctor or mental health professional, particularly in the first few months or if there is any increase in concerning symptoms.

Catherine (Sean's mum): Sean had an assessment with a psychiatrist who diagnosed him as mild to moderately depressed. He was very withdrawn and spending a lot of time in his room. But I did feel hopeful because the psychiatrist said they were going to start him on an antidepressant for a 12-month stint. It took a long time to see any benefit – I would say six to eight weeks before we saw a glimpse of the old Sean. He was fine about taking it. He wanted to get better. We were hanging out for this to work.

- Antidepressants are not addictive.
- Antidepressants do not alter a person's personality. It is the illness, not the medicine, that makes a person 'not like their usual self'.
- It is extremely important that a young person who is taking antidepressant medication is regularly monitored by their doctor, particularly in the first few months.
- Risk of suicide must be assessed for any young person with depression.
- The health professional should discuss with the young person and family a plan to monitor and manage any concerns.
- Support in the form of therapy, information or connection should be put in place for the young person and the family through this time.

24.
Anti-anxiety medication

Elliot: Anti-anxiety medication is used very differently to anti-depressants. The evidence-based treatment of choice for anxiety is psychological therapy. It's about learning to manage your own anxiety. It takes time and practice, but it's really effective.

There isn't a pill that cures anxiety; rather, there are medications that can be used for the acute management of anxiety: they are called anxiolytics. They can have a very fast effect, and give what people are begging for when they're anxious – which is some relief. They relax you and help you go to sleep.

The problem is they can cause both a physiological and a psychological dependence, so if you're using them every day for two weeks you may get a degree of dependence. That's OK, you can wean yourself off them, but it's important to bear in mind that they are tools to use as you learn to manage the illness and its symptoms. These are drugs that should only be used in the short term in anxiety disorders.

Lyndy Matthews (psychiatrist): A severely anxious or depressed young person should initially be seen by a doctor or other health professional every two weeks, or at least every month. In general, the treatment of choice for depression or anxiety will be a talking therapy. Therapy may include family or just be one to one. Some young people will be helped by medication as well. When someone is diagnosed as having a more longstanding or severe condition, studies show that they will do best with a combination of therapy and drugs.

Medications used to treat anxiety and depression fall broadly into two categories:

Antidepressants, which are not addictive, take four to six weeks to have a full effect. The most commonly used is fluoxetine at a dose from 20 to 40mg in the morning.

Anti-anxiety drugs can be prescribed to people with acute anxiety disorders. This is only a short-term treatment (a few weeks), usually while therapy gets under way, as these drugs can cause dependence and interfere with thinking (attention and short-term memory). Anti-anxiety drugs may also be prescribed when someone starts taking an antidepressant, as antidepressants are generally stimulants. The stimulant effect can make people more anxious for the first couple of weeks. The anti-anxiety drugs can help manage symptoms, sleep and any side-effects while the body acclimatises to the antidepressants.

You should definitely ask how long the medication will be continued, how often it will be reviewed, and how it will be tapered off.

- Studies have shown that psychological therapy is the best way of treating anxiety.
- Anti-anxiety medications – anxiolytics – are used very differently to antidepressants. The have an immediate effect, relaxing the person and helping them go to sleep.
- Anti-anxiety medication can cause both physiological and psychological dependence, so these drugs should only be used in the short term.
- Be vigilant about repeat prescriptions for anti-anxiety drugs in the absence of regular review by your doctor.

25.
Tolerating distress

Elliot: A big maintaining factor for depression in some people – that is, the thing that keeps the depression going – is distress intolerance: *I don't like this feeling. I want it to go away now.* They get so distressed that they won't take ownership of their own recovery. They want someone else to fix them: *give me the medication, I'll take it – I want to feel better now.*

An important aspect of therapy is that we're trying to teach our clients to tolerate discomfort, to be able to tolerate unpleasant moods, and not to be afraid of them – because they're going to come, but they're also going to go. Once someone is well I always say to them: 'The good news is you're well again; the bad news is that bad things are going to happen again and you might feel bad again – that's life. So we really need to have a plan in place to deal with that.'

Kirsty: Distress intolerance brings a lot of risk for young people. For instance, if there is a relationship break-up, they feel this devastating sense of rejection. It's such an awful feeling for a young person to have, especially if they really liked the other person. Nowadays, that rejection can be accompanied by all the humiliation that social media can exacerbate: the other person might spread stuff about them, photos that had been private; or they might have to see pictures of the other person on Facebook with someone else.

Such rejection and humiliation can feel intolerable – and that's when the risk of suicide increases, too. It's a way to end those feelings, because at that moment it seems like those feelings will never end. The way young people's brains work means they can have difficulty seeing future possibilities.

With therapy, though, we can help people understand those feelings and how to deal with them. We can help them to see it through, with the support of people around them. It's learning about life, and learning how to foster hope. Bad things happen, but we can ride the storms and come out the other side.

For teens with a particularly sensitive temperament, tolerating distress can be a major challenge. Many youth mental health services provide dialectical behaviour therapy (DBT, one of the cognitive behaviour therapies), which has a focus on managing distress as a key part of its treatment.

- Learning how to tolerate distress is an important part of the treatment of depression and preventing relapse.

26.
Finding a therapist

JK: I saw three therapists before I found the one who was right for me. The first suggested ideas I just couldn't relate to. He wanted me to be a volcano and I thought, *I am really going nuts.* The second one was lovely, but too airy-fairy for me. Then the third one was Louise Armstrong, who was very matter of fact, which was what I needed. She could explain it to me in my terms and put it into my life rather than someone else's life, and I think that's really important.

At that time I had a lot of stigma attached to the illness, so I was sneaking around and hoping no one would see me go into these offices. I was really paranoid. But even though it was hard to find the right person, I wasn't scared off. Once I'd reached out, I thought I'd keep going: *I've made this commitment now and I've got to get well.*

If your teen reaches out for help and meets an idiot, they can be turned off and go back into their shell. Keep trying. Put a little bit of thought into what kind of person they are and what you're looking for, and keep trying.

Hannah: By the time I was admitted to hospital I'd seen two psychologists and two GPs and a dietician and a psychiatrist. I hadn't really connected with any of them. But then I met this doctor at the hospital, and for some reason I really trusted her and I felt she spoke to me in a language I understood. And I felt safe, because up till then I'd been secretly . . . although on the surface I was saying I was fine, I was terrified.

Elliot: Therapy is about understanding the illness in your own context – your triggers, what's keeping it going for you, what to watch out for and so on. It will also help you identify strategies that greatly reduce the impact of depression on your life.

Getting a diagnosis of depression or anxiety tells the professional people what a person has in common with other people who have been diagnosed with depression or anxiety. But everyone's illness is different, and that's why an individual assessment is very important. We want to know why this particular person is presenting in this way at this time, what's keeping it going for them, where their strengths are. That could be quite different from one person to another, even though they've got the same label: depressive disorder, panic disorder, social phobia, whatever.

Kirsty: While there's some similarity in how people may present, the contributing causes can differ quite considerably. That's why there's a risk when someone goes to their GP and gets put on medication but doesn't do anything else to manage their illness. The risk of relapse is greater because none of the other work – identifying potential contributors, perpetuating factors or protective factors – has taken place.

That's where therapy comes in.

When you're choosing a therapist, one of the crucial things to look for is that your young person makes a good personal connection with the therapist. That's going to be the make or break. You may think that they're great and they tick all the boxes, but if the young person hasn't connected, they won't be open with them, and they won't remain engaged with them for long enough to be effective.

The relationship between the therapist and the client accounts for a reasonable chunk of the success of therapy. The better the relationship, the better the chances of good outcomes. One of the roles a parent has in this whole process is modelling attitudes and behaviours to the young person. So yes, the young person needs to know that this is so important that you're going to get them someone they can connect with. You might need to demonstrate the adult wisdom that relationships and trust take time. For instance, you might say to your young person: 'Just one session? Perhaps you could give them a bit more time' (unless there is an obvious problem, such as incompetence or inappropriate behaviour by the therapist).

Listen to what concerns your young person may have about therapy and the therapist. If appropriate, encourage them to share these concerns with the therapist. It's part of the therapist's role to work at engaging with the young person. If the young person is resistant or unsure, you might say: 'How about you try a couple of sessions to get to know them and how they work. Maybe let them know some of the concerns you have, and we can see if that works for you. We can revisit what the options might be from there.' A good therapist should be saying something like that, too: 'Let's have a couple of sessions and see if you're comfortable with me and you feel that we can work well together.'

If it doesn't work with that first therapist, rather than saying, 'We've tried therapy and it didn't work,' look around for someone else they might be more comfortable with. We appreciate this can be challenging to do, as there aren't always other options, but finding a good match is really important.

Important things to look for in a therapist are: good listening abilities; that they take a balanced view of things; that they are careful and comprehensive; that they are reliable; that they have good boundaries.

As a parent you could expect to be given some written information about the therapist's role and the job they do. I would want to know that they were mindful of risk issues, and were thorough enough to be doing risk assessments. Also, that they assess for strengths, seeking out those protective factors within the young person – 'What are you good at? What are you like? What are your interests?' – all those sorts of things. And asking the family about those things as well.

Elliot: I always check back at the end of every session: 'Do you feel like we're heading in the right direction? Does it feel like we're on track? Is there anything you didn't like about today's session? Did you feel uncomfortable about anything I said? Was there anything that you found particularly helpful and that really worked for you?' This helps create a sense of collaboration and ensures the client is being heard and that their needs are being met.

It can be hard for kids to answer, but giving me feedback is something they get better at as we go along. I definitely think it's important for a therapist to open up the possibilities for those conversations. Often people with anxiety and depression have difficulty asserting themselves. They internalise a lot of stuff. So I say, 'This is a win–win for you because you get to give me feedback so that I can make the therapy as good for you as it can possibly be – and also, you get to practise giving feedback. And if you tell me you're not happy with me, that's fantastic – that's a win!' You've got to have fun with it like that.

Kirsty: It's to do with the therapist's connection with the young person as well, opening the door on that kind of conversation. The first few times might be 'yeah', 'nah', 'fine' – you know, the typical adolescent monosyllabic response – but as they get to know you and get more comfortable with your responses to things, then they'll be more inclined to say, 'Well, initially I found it really useful, but now I feel we're just going back over the same stuff and I'm not learning anything new . . .' So that might change over time, and the therapist needs to be open to the young person's point of view.

If the connection isn't great and there aren't other options for a therapist, brainstorm with your young person about the things that might be useful in the therapeutic relationship or process. It might be that they go there to get some information and learn some strategies and techniques, but you look at other options for support they can relate to through youth group leaders or mentors. And as with the medication/therapy issue, its not *either* therapy with a therapist *or* support from mentors/youth workers/guidance counsellors and so on. Both together can be a powerful combination. One caution, though, is to make sure that messages from the two sources are not conflicting. This is why it can be really helpful for a therapist to have the teen's consent to liaise with others involved in their care.

The exciting thing nowadays is that therapy doesn't need to be a face-to-face meeting with someone. There is growing evidence for what are called 'e-therapies' – online programmes that provide the core components of therapy for people. In New Zealand, there is an increasing number of options for this kind of online support, particularly for young people with mild to moderate depression. A great example of this is SPARX – an amazing, New Zealand-developed online game that helps young people learn skills to deal with feeling down, depressed or stressed. It has been found to decrease symptoms of depression and anxiety in young people with mild to moderate depression, as well as in young Maori, young people in alternative education, and young same-sex or both-sex attracted youth. E-therapy options such as this are really exciting, as they increase the availability of therapeutic tools for young people – particularly those who are hesitant to go and talk to a therapist, or who don't have access to one.

JK: I'm a big supporter of SPARX. We need to be aware that young people need tools and steps and pathways to get through problems that are part of the growing-up process and that can seem like very big issues. SPARX gives them a practical way to go through those steps – plus, it's lots of fun. It's an avatar-based computer game – what kid doesn't love to play games on their computer?

Kirsty: Other New Zealand-based e-supports include JK's The Journal, which may be suitable for older adolescents; and thelowdown, which contains information and direct links to online support staff whom young people can text or email for support. Web addresses for these are in the Resources section at the back of the book.

- In the long term, psychological therapy leads to a greatly reduced chance of relapse.
- No matter how good a therapist looks 'on paper', it's crucial that your young person makes a good personal connection with them.
- Give each therapist at least a couple of sessions to see if they are going to be a good match, but if they're not, don't give up on therapy. Look around for someone your young person feels more comfortable with. It's frustrating, but worth it.
- There are some great online resources for support, including e-therapy through SPARX.

27.
How involved should parents be?

Adrienne (Marly's mum): I got this phone call from the school counsellor: 'We've got Marly here and we're worried. We think she might try and hurt herself.' I got to the school as quickly as I could. It turned out Marly, who was 15, had been going to the school counselling service for five weeks. Five weeks! I said to the counsellor, 'And you didn't think to involve us?' And then I said to Marly: 'Did you not want us involved?' She looked confused, and it turned out she hadn't even been asked.

If they'd asked her and she'd said she didn't want us involved, fine. But the automatic thought was, *let's not include the family*. That's the default setting. I have no difficulties about counsellors who feel unable to engage the parents because the child refuses. But counsellors who don't even ask, and don't find out what the situation is with the parents in detail and don't look for the benefits . . . I think it's terrible.

Kirsty: It's vital that parents are included in their young person's care. They are the ones who are responsible for the young person, they're with them a significant chunk of the time, they can make the difference as to whether things progress or not, and most importantly they can be a significant support for the young person.

However, therapists can hold different points of view about parental involvement; and some do not include any parents. This is something to ask about and to be clear about in your initial encounter with the therapist. It can also depend on the context in which the young person is seeing a therapist (for instance, through school or church or the mental health system). The reality is, though, that parents need to be included. They need to be educated about what is happening for their young person and how they can best support them. What this inclusion looks like, however, may be different to what the parents want and expect: they may end up having far less – or sometimes far more – involvement than they had anticipated.

With teenagers, consent and confidentiality become big issues, and this is often quite hard for parents to accept. Particularly for older adolescents, part of what is going on for them may mean that they don't want a lot of parental involvement, and that can be immensely difficult for parents.

I'm sure most parents will be either uncertain or frustrated when a health professional says, 'I can't talk to you about this because I don't have your son or daughter's consent.' It's a grey area. However, to be of any help, the primary relationship has to be between the therapist and the adolescent: the adolescent needs to trust that what they say is confidential. Usually clinicians will err on the side of preserving the trust and the relationship with the client, balancing off against the safety of the client and keeping them well.

Young people should be told something along the lines of: 'What you talk to me about in this room is confidential. This means that I won't tell anyone about it unless you agree to that, although the professional team I am part of will be kept up to date with what is going on so we can work together to support you. [Who is in this team will depend on the setting, but needs to be stated to the young person.] The only time I would break this confidentiality is if I was concerned about your safety – if you were going to hurt yourself or someone else, or were at risk of hurt from others. If that was the case I would talk with you about who we would need to tell to keep you safe and how we would do that.'

Confidentiality does not need to mean no parental involvement. In the first instance, particularly for a young adolescent, you should be part of the initial interviews identifying what is going on. Remember, however, that if the therapist does see you separately (that is, without your young person present), what you say to them may not remain confidential. They may need to be able to talk with the young person about what you have talked about if it is relevant to their treatment, otherwise it's difficult for them to maintain their connection, engagement and trust. Remember, they are your child's therapist, not yours.

With an older adolescent you may see very little of their therapist. It's very difficult when you're aware that the young person has a particular perspective on you and the family, and you're thinking, *that's all the therapist will be hearing, just one side of the story. They'll get it all wrong!* But again, that's about trusting the professional to be able to sift through all that. That's part of their role, to get the young person to a place where their thinking is clearer, where it's more fact than opinion-based. Part of that might involve checking in with you, or it might not.

> Although we know that a loving and well-functioning family is a key factor that protects against depression while family discord is a risk factor, the best way to involve parents and families in interventions is surprisingly unclear.—Gluckman Report, p. 200

The issue of ongoing parental involvement in the adolescent therapy process is a really sensitive and sometimes painful one for parents. It is very unlikely that you will be sitting in all the sessions with your young person, or that you will be told all the areas that they are working on with the therapist. Of course, it depends on the age of the young person – there's quite a difference between an 18-year-old and a 12- to 13-year-old. Part of the therapy process will involve negotiation and discussion around bringing the parents in, in whatever way is deemed most useful.

If the adolescent is younger, you really need a therapist who will be having some ongoing contact with you. It could be that every three or four sessions they have 15 minutes or so where you all sit in the room and the therapist might say, 'These are the sorts of things we're working on. It feels like we're going really well. These are the things she'd like to feed back to you . . .' This can be quite a structured feedback that identifies key aspects of how the young person is doing, and key things the parent can be doing to support them. It might involve using the terminology they are using in the session to talk about the depression or anxiety; supporting the young person with their therapy 'homework'; or making some shifts or changes in the way things work at home or in your relationship with the young person.

If the therapist recommends changes in relationships at home, part of the treatment for the young person may be family therapy, or some individual parenting work for the parents. Your engagement in this will have a significant impact on the success of the young person's treatment.

If the adolescent is a bit older, say 16 and up, unless you are having family therapy you should assume that you're not going to be very involved with the process. You need to make sure, however, that the therapist is someone you trust, and that they're aware that they can contact you. Let them know your availability and willingness, and that you trust them to contact you if there are concerns about risk. It's awfully hard because you are likely to be quite distant from the process.

Part of their role will also be to encourage the young person to share with you where there are issues you need to be aware of, or things they want you to do to support them. You need to be ready to listen when they are doing this – *listen*, not defend or react. They will typically be sharing something where they are worried about your reaction – that you might be angry, ashamed of them, or disappointed. Be open-minded and calm. Thank them for sharing it with you. Let them know you might need time to process it. Remind them of your love for them. And remember this is all happening in the context of a natural shift in the parent–child relationship anyway. Focus on nurturing the relationship they have with you and finding a way forward.

Lyndy Matthews (psychiatrist): I have worked for 10 years in Maori health, and that has given me so much insight into the fact that no one is truly an individual – we are all part of a family or some other kind of network.

Elliot: The young person's cultural background will also be key in determining the appropriate level of family involvement and who 'family' are. Parents and families need to be involved – part of the therapist's role is finding a way to do this that is going to help both the young person and the family. Of course, all of this also depends on the seriousness of the illness. When a young person needs to be hospitalised or to have more intensive intervention, parental involvement will increase.

When a young person develops a mental illness it can be very stressful for the family, and the challenge of supporting the young person and making decisions about their care can exacerbate existing differences and conflicts. Inclusion of parents and family also obviously becomes more challenging in the context of difficult family relationships, where the family situation is a contributor to the young person's depression. But in many cases this indicates a need for *increased* family involvement (unless the young person is nearing independence), rather than less.

Lyndy Matthews (psychiatrist): The sorts of scenarios where people legitimately don't want their families involved are where they have a very dysfunctional family, often where alcohol is a significant factor; where they can't predict the response; where they may get blamed or attacked for seeking help, for bringing the family's business into a public domain. But even in this kind of scenario, we can usually work with them to the point where someone will emerge as a support.

Kirsty: In blended families there can be queries about who the most appropriate adults are to be involved in decisions around a young person's care. Professionals need to be aware of who all the important people are, and the role they have played or currently play. Part of the therapeutic journey may include people who haven't been present in the young person's life for some time, and this can bring considerable challenges for the adults. Ensure that the professionals are aware of any challenges that might add further stress on the young person.

How involved should parents be?

- Family is usually a vital part of a young person's recovery, but the process the young person goes through with their therapist is confidential.
- Remember, they are your child's therapist, not yours. The therapist's primary relationship is with the young person, and they need to guard their relationship and the trust they have with the young person.
- The level of parental involvement will depend on the age of the young person, the severity of their illness, their cultural background and the type of therapy being received. This is something you can ask about in your initial encounter.
- All families can be involved in supporting and assisting their young person in their recovery. Ask what that could mean in your case, and be open-minded about what this may involve.

28.
Different kinds of therapy

Helene: My GP referred me to a mental health clinic and I saw a psychiatrist who put me on antidepressants, and a clinical psychologist whose field was CBT [cognitive behaviour therapy] and I found it very helpful. She said something that I really related to: she'd been crossing the road and she felt like everyone was looking at her and thinking things about her. That was really eye-opening for me. As a young person myself, the world seemed so huge and I thought everyone must be noticing what I was doing and thinking about it and being critical – but really no one is paying you much attention at all. So for me it was so good to challenge those automatic assumptions – to stop and ask, *is that realistic?* And she offered me strategies, like imagining a protective bubble around myself.

It was so helpful to know that other people have similar experiences, because I had always felt I wasn't normal. *What's wrong with me?* Now I understand that people simply don't show their difficulties to the outside world. You look at other people and think, *why can't I be like that? They look happy all the time*. So I was always measuring myself against other people, thinking that only I had these problems.

Effective Treatments for Depression and Anxiety: The Psychological Therapies

What are psychological therapies?

There are many psychological therapies used by therapists of one sort or another to treat anxiety and depression. They usually involve spoken conversation (which is why they are sometimes referred to as 'talk therapies') between therapist and patient (or 'client'). The conversations in psychological therapies address the problems and concerns the person is experiencing, and through this bring about improvements in the person's mental health and wellbeing. The various therapies are based on different psychological theories and use different techniques to help bring about change.

It is important to know that not all of the psychological therapies are 'evidence-based'. Evidence-based treatments have been shown to be effective in scientific studies. Just as medication can bring about changes in brain functioning, reducing symptoms of anxiety and depression, so can effective psychological therapies. So, as well as teaching helpful ways to cope, good therapy may literally 'rewire' your brain. The following psychological therapies have an evidence base for justifying their use in teens who have anxiety or depression.

Cognitive behaviour therapies

The cognitive behaviour therapies (CBTs) are a 'family' of therapies that share the same psychological theories around developing and maintaining mental health problems. These theories emphasise the role of learning – both through the responses and contexts we experience around our behaviour (conditioning) and through our observations of others as we grow up (social learning). They also emphasise the influence of unhelpful beliefs and thinking styles that people can develop in association with their life experiences.

The different CBTs use techniques based on these theories to break down the unhelpful processes that keep a person's problems going (the *maintaining factors*). These techniques generally fall into two categories: 'behavioural' strategies (experimenting with doing things differently to find more helpful, effective ways of coping); and 'cognitive' strategies (helping the person develop more healthy, helpful ways of thinking to combat the negative thinking so typical of depression, and the catastrophic, fearful thinking of anxiety). There is also a big emphasis in the CBTs on learning 'adaptive' skills (such as problem-solving and communication skills) that a person can take forward in their life following therapy and recovery, to keep themselves well in the future.

The CBTs have the most extensive evidence base justifying their use for treating depression and anxiety in both adults and adolescents.

Psychodynamic therapies

The psychodynamic model argues that psychological problems result from problematic unconscious thoughts and feelings. They are 'unconscious' in the sense that we protect ourselves from the anxiety they provoke using 'defences' (such as 'repressing' thoughts or feelings from awareness) to keep them away. By becoming aware of this unconscious material, and dealing with it, the person's symptoms and problems may resolve. A psychodynamic therapist helps a person gain that awareness and move forward in their life.

There is clear evidence for psychodynamic therapies being effective for the treatment of some mental disorders in adults. However, there is less published research on their effectiveness in treating depression and anxiety in adolescents.

Interpersonal therapy

Interpersonal therapy (IPT) says that the context of someone's depression or anxiety – their significant relationships – needs to be the key focus. It argues that depression and anxiety affect and are affected by those relationships. In IPT the goal of treatment is to reduce symptoms and improve relationships. In practice this begins by identifying problem areas in the client's life and relationships. The therapist then helps the client develop skills and techniques to apply to these problem areas, thereby improving the relationships.

IPT has a strong evidence base in the treatment of mental disorder in adults (especially for depression), and a developing evidence base for treating depression and anxiety disorders in adolescents.

Family therapies

Family therapies focus on the role that relationships within a family may have on a teenager's mental health problems. They involve the whole family meeting with the therapist with a view to gaining insights around the way the family is functioning. The aim is to then develop more helpful communication patterns and relationships.

Family therapies may be effective where the family dynamics have a contribution to the problem, but where there are broader problems for the teen – which is often the case in adolescent anxiety and depression – they would likely also require individual treatment.

Online therapies

It is increasingly acknowledged that there may never be enough adequately qualified mental health professionals to meet treatment needs in the community using the traditional face-to-face therapy model. In response to this, efforts have been made to develop treatment programmes that can be delivered online as a form of self-help. Some of these programmes have an evidence base, with best-practice guidelines tending to endorse those based on CBT principles. Some have been developed specifically for teens, such as SPARX here in New Zealand. These typically involve working through a series of lessons or modules, and incorporate a 'helpline' that allows you to contact people for additional assistance if this is needed.

How long does psychological therapy take?

The length of psychological therapy varies, depending largely on how complex the teenager's depression or anxiety might be. Having said this, psychodynamic therapies tend to be longer than most CBTs and IPT. Both CBT and IPT for depression or anxiety might be expected to involve at least 10 sessions (though potentially many more than this) of weekly to fortnightly hour-long meetings with the therapist. However, there are briefer applications of CBT, and some people may get substantial benefit from even four to six sessions.

Other factors influencing outcomes

Research shows that the therapist has a significant effect on outcomes, beyond the type of therapy they are delivering. This is thought to be because of the inherently personal nature of therapy, and the understandable importance of factors such as therapist empathy, trustworthiness, genuineness and capacity for attentive listening. The other obvious therapist factor is their competence: an evidence-based therapy would not be expected to work if delivered by a therapist not competent in that therapy.

29. Matching resources to world view

Elliot: It's important that any treatment works within the appropriate world view of the individual. This is important right throughout the process – from initial assessment, how the four Ps are considered (see page 73), what the goals of treatment are, and who is involved in treatment.

Not being able to find a clinician from the same world view can be a major barrier for some families seeking treatment. There are Maori and Pasifika services available now, but unfortunately not enough. If none are available to you, it's important to ask how any therapist will take *who you are* into account in terms of the therapy process, in their understanding of the young person and in treatment goals. In terms of process, with Maori for example, it might include giving time for whakawhanaungatanga (acknowledging whakapapa); offering space for karakia at the beginning and end of sessions; and using the powhiri process as a guide to session structure. It might be about recognition of the broader role of whanau in the healing process. Or it may be in the types of therapy that are offered or the models used to conceptualise what is going on, and what recovery might look like – for example, how spirituality, belonging and broader whanau are considered as part of the picture for the young person.

- Ask how any therapist will take *who you are* into account in terms of the therapy process, in their understanding of the young person, and in treatment goals.
- It's important that any treatment works within the appropriate world view of the individual, whether that's because of ethnicity, age or any other reason.
- There are not enough specialty services, so check how the available services can meet your needs.

30.
Step by step

Kirsty: Often a client will come in for an initial consultation and they will say things like: 'I just want my life back.' Or 'I want to be back in school.' Or, more likely, their parents will say, 'He just has to get back to school.'

The thing about goals like this is that they are *end goals*; and at that moment, when the young person is so depressed and anxious, they seem impossible. So in a way, naming these end goals can feed the hopelessness they're already feeling.

As a therapist you serve your client by keeping that end goal in mind, but breaking it down into much smaller, simpler, achievable goals. So with the broad 'getting back to school' goal, a good therapist would work proactively with the school to get the young person back and engaged. This might mean a first goal of meeting with the school principal and school guidance counsellor to talk about what options there might be; then getting the young person to school three mornings a week, then two days and three mornings – a very staggered approach where they're being dropped off and met, monitored throughout the day, and a lot of care is being taken to get the balance right between feeling overwhelmed and continuing to move forward. The small goals feed into the overarching goal of getting their life back. That's where hope comes in: *I can't go back to school yet, but I can do that. I can go to a meeting.*

Elliot: A goal that's clear and feasible is attractive, and when it's achieved it increases confidence. By contrast, a goal like *being part of that social group again* may not be clear enough; or *being able to go into that shopping mall without having a panic attack* may not be realistic very early in treatment. These would risk setting up your teen for failure. And they really *feel* perceived failure. But perhaps what they can do is go for a walk down the shopping street of the suburb at a time when there are not a lot of people around; then they can go with their best friend on a Tuesday night when it's not very busy. They can take those steps and their confidence grows.

We mentioned this before and it's a really important point: recovery is rarely straight. For some, it can be like a rollercoaster. The expectations of both the young person and the parents need to be realistic. That way each step can be celebrated. Part of the process of learning how to move forward is getting the young person and their family members to be aware of the sort of things that impact both internally and externally on how treatment might progress. It's about everyone hanging in there together and supporting each other through the process.

The rest of this book looks at this: What can parents do to walk alongside their young person, to stand by them?

- End goals such as 'I want my life back' can seem overwhelming and impossible.
- A therapist will break those end goals into manageable steps so that the person will gain a sense of achievement along the way, and build confidence.
- Recovery is rarely in a straight line – there will likely be good weeks and bad weeks. Be realistic in expectations, and celebrate all steps forward along the way.

PART FOUR

Holding The Hope

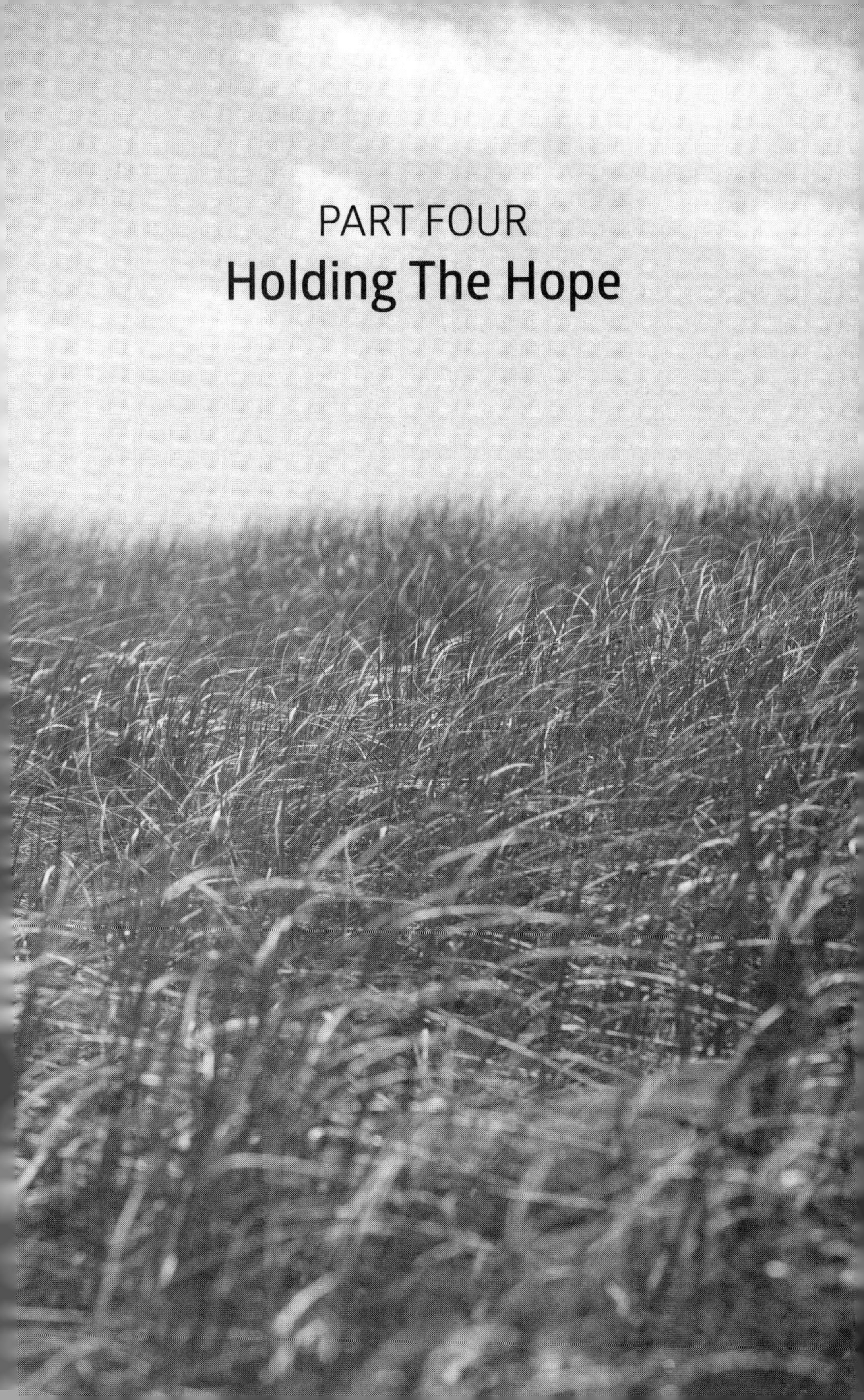

31.
Hope

JK: Hope is the knowledge that things can and will get better. Depression is an absence of hope, and that is the horror that lies at its heart. When I was depressed I didn't have any hope, and so I needed others to carry the hope for me. For me, it was Michael Jones telling me, 'You've got a good heart, JK' – it seems like a little thing, but I hung onto it. It represented hope – hope that I wasn't as bad as I feared; hope that I could be a good person, and that that was worth living for.

I believe there's a tonne of hope in the stories we share with each other about the tough times we've been through. I offer you my story – that I've been to hell but I came back again – and it's my offering of hope to those who are currently in that awful place.

You could be a parent, a friend, a youth worker – doesn't matter. But when someone you care about has forgotten who they are and has no hope for the future, you can remind them who they are: that they are a good person, that they have a future, even if they can't see it right now. You can hold the hope for them.

Levi: From when I was 14 or 15, I lived under a bridge for a year and I experienced the life of a homeless man, drinking every day, having no money but asking with my hand out, 'Do you have a dollar for the bus?' In that world of mine it was all individual, every man for himself.

Now I know that got me nowhere, that every-man-for-himself way of being. I believe we should all help each other. I believe that we aren't called to be sole operators; we're called to be a community of people who help each other. There's so much poverty, and so many kids who don't have support.

And it's that support that finally got me to where I am right now – from Matt Grey, who is now the manager at ZEAL youth centre. If it wasn't for his faith and strength and courage and consistency, I would not be the person I am today. I was on my way to jail – a friend and I had done three aggravated robberies and I had breached my bail three times. But Matt came to court and said he would mentor me, and that I could move in with him and his family, and the judge said, 'You've got one more chance to do things right.'

That made me break down and cry because that was my prayer – that I wouldn't go to jail and that I would have family who would love and care for me, and that I would change my life. I didn't want to be this gangster out on the street with no sense of belonging. I wanted something that was stable.

After that, I was on 24-hour curfew, and in three months my life had completely changed.

It flicked my whole life around. I started talking to people, I was happy, I had this sense of belonging, and the world went brighter and brighter and brighter. I wanted to help people. One day I spent all the money I had and I made sandwiches, and I went out and gave them to the homeless people. It felt good to do good. I started giving to people. It was not about me. I want to give back to the people because of what the community of people around me gave to me.

It's so hard to not know who you are. I was constantly trying to find out who I was – am I a street kid, an alcoholic? But I was just a kid looking for love. I was looking in the wrong places. It was false love. For 16 years of my life I didn't know what was good love, till I met Matt.

So I didn't get hope from my parents or my family in the normal sense. But now Matt and his wife and kids are my family, and my family is here at ZEAL, and in the community that's around me. That's what gives me hope.

32.
Keep trying

Kirsty: As parents, as our children grow older and our relationship with them changes, we often don't feel confident – and this is amplified in the context of mental health. We might be getting very minimal response from our teen, and we can assume we've said or done the wrong thing. We often don't know until later what the outcome of our actions will be.

There's no silver bullet when it comes to teenage mental illness, but there are options, and the most important message of all is: keep trying. That has come through clearly in the conversations we've had with young people who have recovered from mental illness. They've talked about how, even if it didn't necessarily feel it was helping at the time, the fact that their parents were there and trying was in itself a protective factor. As they started to come out from their depression they could see that it brought some hope, knowing someone was there.

So: your presence, your questions, your checking in, most importantly your listening, is evidence that you care and that you tried. Even if you did get it quite wrong at times, you did the right thing by being there.

Hannah: I understand that it can be hard to know how to ask, especially if the young person doesn't give much of an answer. I guess, for me, one of the hard things was that I didn't know what anything was. I thought everybody felt like I did – that life was just really hard. So if you feel there's not something right with your kid, rather than trying to do the talking yourself, get professional help sooner rather than later. Kids don't know what it is they need from their parents. But maybe what we need from parents is them having the knowledge to normalise, to say, 'Some people have this, this or this; that's something that lots of people have.'

Elliot: I think it's useful to think of depression as a disorder of hope. It's often experienced as a state of *hopelessness*. Inherent in the condition is this negative expectation, this pessimism. It's so important for all of us – health professionals, family, friends – to factor that into our encounters with someone who is experiencing depression. They aren't going to give you a big smile and say, 'Wow, that was really useful, thanks Mum, of course it's going to get better, I can see that now!' If you suggest something, they may well say it sucks. Suggest they give it a go anyway, to see what happens. It's usually not as bad as expected.

Kirsty: I think of it like this: what you're doing is standing by them, and you're holding the hope that they are not able to hold for themselves. You're standing by them despite what you might be getting back from them (which may often be very little).

It's sort of the difficult, extreme edge of parenting, isn't it? You might be getting little response, you might be getting lack of engagement, either with you or with the therapeutic people that you're trying to set in place. But that doesn't mean that what you're doing isn't purposeful and helping. It's just that it's really hard in that moment to see it.

Your young person may take very small steps back to wellness – so small that, as parents, we don't even know they're taking them. Our interview with Jacob showed this. Over the years of his depression, while his parents had seen little difference in his behaviour, there were shifts going on internally. They continued to worry that he might commit suicide, as he had tried to once before. In fact, Jacob's thinking had moved a long way from that, but they weren't aware of it because it was an internal shift for him.

Sometimes the depression behaviour shifts more into normal adolescent behaviour. What's observed can still look similar – they may still seem withdrawn and distant – but there are subtle changes:

now they're listening to music and texting their friends when they are in their room all the time, rather than sleeping, crying and being preoccupied with morbid thoughts.

- Even if you do get it wrong at times, you're doing the right thing by being there and trying.
- When someone is depressed they might not be able to show they appreciate your efforts, but your efforts show you care, and that is very important.
- Shifts will happen internally for the young person on their path to wellbeing that won't always be noticeable. Watch for the subtle changes.

33.
I believe in you

Matt (Levi's new dad): Levi gets in ruts – I term it the black dog. You can see it consume him: *I'm really sad and I don't know why*. I think there's a real struggle inside him, and I know he gets frustrated. He feels like his life has turned around, so he shouldn't still feel those things.

I don't have pearls of wisdom: I just sit there with him and let him talk, and let him just be sad. It's really important to say to him, 'Well, of course, bro, that makes sense, you don't just get over things. You're kind of ripped off in your early life and that's going to be a struggle for a long time and that's going to have some effects. You can't beat yourself up about that. It is what it is.' That's probably all I really say. The rest of the time I just sit outside with him and have a cup of coffee and don't say much. Just be there with him.

A lot of counsellors talk about this dance between validation and change talk that the caregiver can do, in our conversations with young people who are struggling. Acknowledging their experience, that whole, 'I understand what you're saying, and god that sounds so hard.' You can't live in that, because nothing would ever change; but you can't go straight to, 'OK, you've got a problem with that and you need to do this and this and this.' Then they're like, 'But you don't understand, you don't get it. You don't get how this actually feels.' So there has to be a balance between the two.

The person has to be understood, and to know that you're really there with them; and then you can gently guide them. And anyone can do that. Not just counsellors. Any caregiver or parent.

Kirsty: That dance between validation and change talk is so vitally important, and quite a shift for some parents. It's so easy to shift straight into parent mode – having the answers (or pretending you have them) and informing the young person what they need to do. Any suggestions around change are going to fall on deaf ears, however, if they think you don't *get* them; if you're not hearing how things are for them. This can also add to the pressure, as the suggestions for change feel like just one more thing they aren't getting right.

Scarlet: Parents should accept and understand who you are, but also the environment around you and what influences you're under. Then they can understand why you might be feeling that way, and give you time to figure out stuff. Not judge you, pretty much.

Kirsty: Listen to them, give them space, and try to understand. You won't always be able to do this – their world is different from the one you grew up in and sometimes it just won't make sense. But at the very least, you can empathise that they are going through a really rough time at the moment. That bit – the difficult emotions bit – you can probably relate to, even if you can't relate to what's causing it. Try and find something in what they are distressed about that makes sense, something to relate to and validate, even if the whole thing is difficult to understand or immensely frustrating. You can say, 'I can see how, when you are having such constant low thoughts about yourself, going out must be really hard and feel quite scary and overwhelming' – even if you don't agree with those thoughts or understand why they are so stuck on them.

Here are some useful things to think about when validating. As a parent this can be a hard way to respond to a young person: it's a shift, and it takes time and practice.

- Give them time to talk, and listen without interrupting or judging them. Sit down with them, take some extra minutes to give them time, and show by your actions that you are taking them seriously.
- Summarise what they have said to you (again without judgment and your own bits added in), acknowledging and

capturing the feelings or emotions behind what they are saying.
- Look for a way their actions or emotions make sense given their current situation or their history, and name and validate that.
- Be yourself, be real, acknowledge the challenges in this: 'This is awkward and I'm really not sure I'm getting it, but I want to try and I want you to know that despite me getting frustrated I get that this is going on for you and it's really hard.'
- Take the opportunity to acknowledge the strengths in the person, to provide them with the hope. 'I can see it's hard, and you know what, I've seen you get through some hard stuff before. That other time, you really showed how strong you can be. This may take time and feel a lot bigger, but in small bits and with us all around you, I know you can do it.'

The more of these validating conversations that take place, the more open the young person is going to be to the change conversations – the ones where you start to talk about the steps they need to take.

The *way* we move from validation to change conversations is also important. If they hear: 'I understand what is going on *and* I wonder if some of the steps your therapist talked about would be useful here. Should we take a look at them and see which ones?', this is likely to have much greater motivational impact than if you tell them: 'I understand what is going on *but* if you just did what your therapist said it would be a lot better.'

In therapy, we talk about using *and* versus *but*: 'I understand, *and* . . .' versus 'I understand, *but* . . .' It's such a small thing, but it can really make you stop and think about what you're saying and, most importantly, how it is going to be received by the young person and motivate them towards change – or not.

The validation and change-talk dance that Matt speaks about is tricky but well worth the effort, because validation helps build hope. *They get it, they understand me, they care about me and they want to help me find ways through.* This is very different from: *they just want me to change; once more I'm not good enough.* Hope empowers change.

34.
'It's going to be all right'

Mel (Hannah's mum): Giving hope is absolutely vital. Full recovery isn't just possible, it's non-negotiable. It's going to happen. And it's about giving people that hope when they're saying 'I'm in a hole and someone's putting the cover over me and it's so dark and so awful I can't imagine coming out of it.'

As a parent, what worked for me was remaining really positive, remaining Hannah's light. I'd say: 'I know that must be awful.' You've got to choose your words carefully because they'll shout back, 'You don't know!' 'Well, no, I don't know, but I can see how awful it is for you and I want to tell you that you're going to get better.' 'I will never get better!' 'I know it feels like that, but you will. And I am really excited about your future. Now, did you see in the news today that the prime minister said blah blah, blah . . .'

You've got to manage the discussion. Don't have a discussion with the depression or the anxiety or the eating disorder. 'I'm interested in you, I'm really excited about your future. Now . . .' 'What's in my future?' *I'll have that discussion!* 'I can see you travelling overseas with your friends after you've got your degree. Now, let's go for a drive.' And when you do these things – driving and chatting – you're really saying, *I'm here and I'm with you and I'll never, ever give up.*

Catherine (Sean's mum): We've never given up hope. Ever. And what's kept us going? At the end of the day, we know Sean is a good person. He has a good heart, a beautiful soul and is extremely loving. All those things have been given to him for a reason. We've told him, with all his wonderful traits and all his experience, he can now go out there and help others. And we think he thinks that, too. As far as this book is concerned, he has said to us that it would be good if he could pass on even one little thing – it would be worth it, in his eyes. Three or four months ago we believe Sean would not have been happy to be part of this project, but he is now, and it's an indication of how much better he's feeling.

Failing to believe that it's going to be alright in the end is simply not an option. If you're going to give up on your child, well, who's there for them? I've always felt from the beginning that we will be alright.

Elliot Taylor (youth worker): It's said that only two things can result in change: willpower or divine intervention. But the role of 'alongsiders' – that is, friends, parents, youth workers or whatever – is that we can awaken the will of that person to make change. Because otherwise there is that position where someone says, *I've got no divine intervention and no will*, so they're kind of hung out to dry. That's the importance of community: we can awaken the will. We can do that by believing in them when they don't believe in themselves – in a sense, telling them or reminding them who they really are. When we believe in someone before they believe in themselves, they can come to believe, too. With my friend, all I did was I announced to her who I believe she is, and I believed 100 percent. And she later said, 'Thank you for seeing me before I saw myself.'

Brook (youth worker): If a kid has a problem and they have to tackle that problem alone, depending on the size of that problem it might be overwhelming. So if I'm with them and I can help them navigate that, it's a shared problem. *Yes, I carry hope for you*, but I would build on that and say: 'Let's share the problem. Is that mental health issue yours, or ours? Is that addiction yours, or is it ours? Is that struggle yours, or is it ours?'

Amitai: I needed others to remind me: 'This is not you.' I saw myself in a pretty negative way at that time. I had no emotional energy and I was very low. I was drinking. I was drunk during my English exam and I failed it – the first exam I'd ever failed. Because of some hard things going on in my family, I was a kid going off the rails and I didn't believe in myself any more. But two teachers said things that kind of stayed with me and probably helped to snap me out of the state I was in, reminding me of who I was: 'This is not you'.

The previous year I had been top of maths in my form and the school had thought, *this guy is going to do wonders*. Then everything crashed and burned. Anyway, this teacher who had always taken an interest in me got me into his office and pulled out the attendance sheet and said, 'Look at this. See all of those black crosses? That's your attendance. At the end of last year you were held as the person that was going to kick some ass, and now all we can see is crosses next to your name. You're better than this.'

At the time I didn't have the emotional energy to make any changes. I didn't tell anybody about what was actually going on. But what he said stayed with me and it made a difference, even though it didn't seem like it at the time.

And my English teacher as well – when I failed the exam she said, 'What is this?' She wasn't willing to accept that this was me now. It stuck with me. It was a glimpse of something that I possibly am, even though I couldn't see it myself.

When you're in that space you don't even want to talk about it. You just think, *how can someone help?* I know that if they'd said, 'Is everything OK?' I would have said, 'Everything's fine.'

I felt like I was going undetected and I liked it like that. It was quite a reality check that people were observing me.

I guess the way they approached me was good, too, because it was like: 'I know what you're capable of, I know what you've done,' which is affirming. Whereas if it had been my parents, the approach would have been: 'What the hell are you doing?' That's just pressure.

35.
Little moments of hope

JK: In depression there's no hope and no enjoyment. But as you start to come out of it you start to remember the things you like. And that's when you take the first steps on the rest of your journey – the journey back to wellness.

Jacob: Even during the worst years, we might go on a holiday, go camping, do a walk along a river, be out in nature with the family. It was something I probably didn't want to go and do, probably hated the idea of, but once I was there . . . I remember walking along a river and everyone's there, and just for a moment you can, not forget the depression, but see what it might be like without it. Little chinks of light. Wherever they come from, those are the helpful little gifts from God.

You do notice that when you're starting to feel better you kind of have these feelings of being light. And happy. I remember at some point just noticing that I'm feeling pretty good and happy with things. And feeling really stoked, and kind of exhausted as you realise that. It's a really good feeling, however long that lasts, and you start taking it for granted.

I find that most of the time for the last two years I've been on an even gradient and I haven't gone up or down too drastically, and that's how I've learned to deal with it. When I'm feeling down I don't think of it as depression any more because I'm not scared of it. It's just feeling sad, and everyone feels sad, and so I can deal with it in that way, and know that the next day will probably be different.

Hannah: The biggest thing is having some sense of hope. In the early stages it's so awful: you literally think, *I'm never going to get out of this, whatever this is*, and it feels impossible.

The hope comes in the little moments that you have, or the

conversations with friends that let you know the real world still exists, that your little cocoon of unhappiness is not normal and it is possible to break out of it.

Hearing other people's stories, how they've come through it: other people have done it, so I can, too. Someone else has eaten two biscuits; I can, too. Everyone else is at the party; I can be there, too. Someone else has recovered from depression and passed all their exams; it can be done.

Sean: A really good thing was meeting people with the same experiences. That was huge. And older people as well. People that I really respected in the music community.

After I left school I got a fulltime job in a music shop, and my boss there was a massive influence. He was my parents' age, but he used to play in our band. We got really close, and hung out a lot outside of work. He'd been through a lot of stuff, and I was lucky enough for him to tell me about it. I respected him so much and think he's a great individual, and still do – but he's gone through a lot worse than I've been through. I guess it gave me a sense of hope that you could come out the other side and be such a great person. That's what it's all about, isn't it?

PART FIVE

The Family Stripped Bare

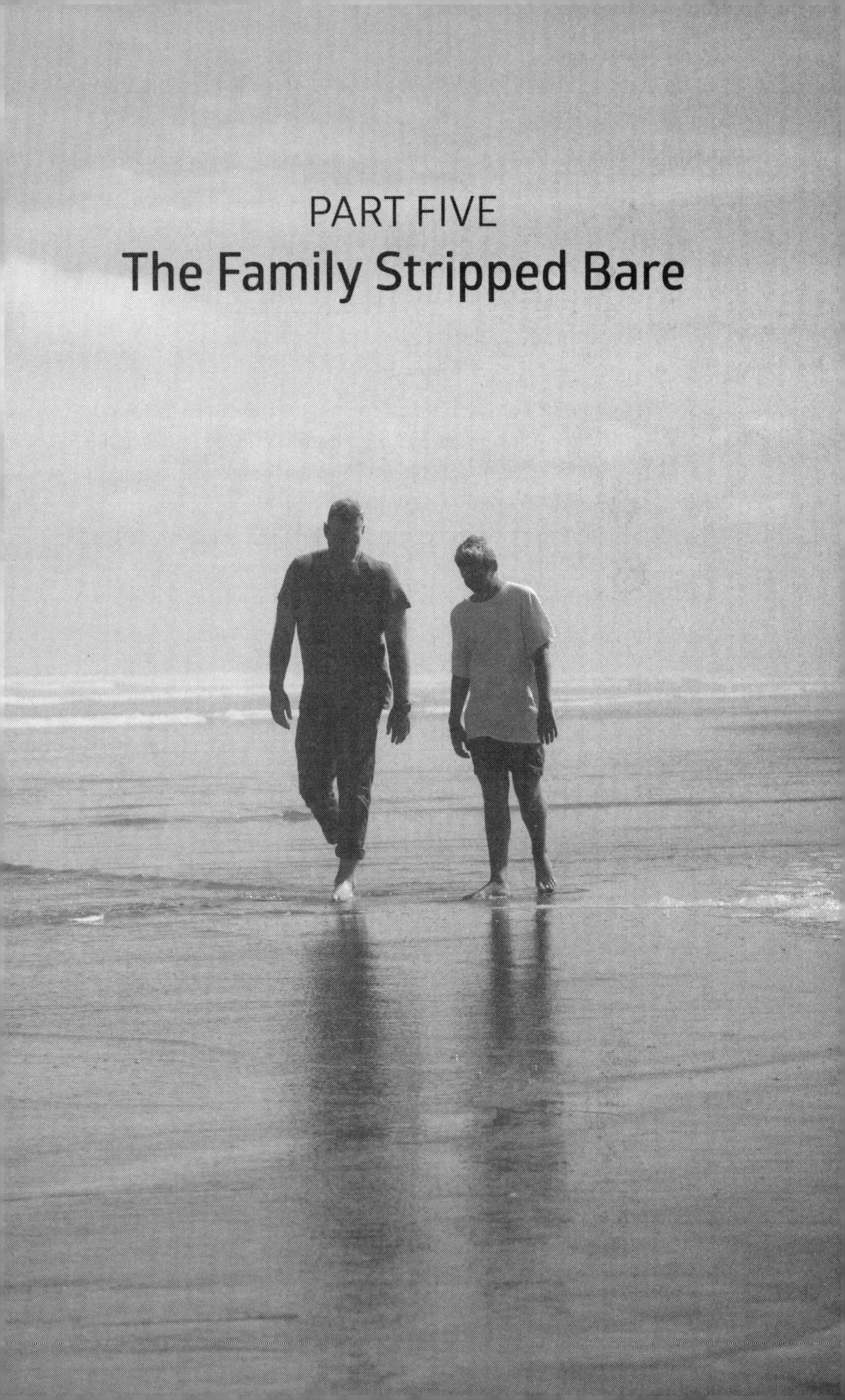

36.
Love the real child

JK: Someone said something interesting to me once – it sounds cold, but it's accurate. I was talking about a friend who'd had a problem with their family, and I said, 'You can't pick your parents.' And this person said, 'Yeah, and you can't pick your kids either.' All you can do is be the best you can be; and love the child you've got.

Layla (Christie's mum): When a child has mental illness, a lot of things that they and you hoped for might no longer be possible. Some of your dreams for your child must die or be put on hold – certainly, they must change. That was really real for us. Christie's sporting prowess is something we as parents have enjoyed – I get a thrill when she wins things – and, of course, that all went away. And I thought, *that's it, she'll never be able to be active again*. And she may not. We may find that now she's back to leading quite an active life she does lose weight again; and for me the choice will be healthy body weight over that level of activity and sporting prowess.

It's an identity thing, and she does enjoy it, it's part of her make-up. But you strip that away, and the child we have is the real child. All the packaging around that is nice to have – the child who wins medals. But it's not what makes them your child. So we did have to confront that. And I'll be honest, I missed that. She had been on the cusp of going off to the next level, competing in other cities, and she couldn't go. Other kids did, and word would filter back, and I'd think, *oh, she should be there, too*. So that's been quite a challenge. It's a grief. You're grieving for what your child is not experiencing, and for what you as a parent are not experiencing, too.

JK: When I had depression I really thought I would never get myself back as a person. I'm quite sure that parents of kids with mental illness fear that they won't get their child back. Be patient. Understand that what they've got is an illness, and with the right help it will pass and they will get better. You will get your child back – although, sure, both they and you will have changed and grown as a result of their experiences.

Elliot: We can't offer a recipe or a formula but we can talk about principles, and this is one of the biggest: try to separate the illness from the person. Never forget about who your child is, and hold on to the wonderful things about them, in spite of the mental health challenges they may have.

Kirsty: I think it's really useful to acknowledge the grieving process that a parent might go through when their child has a mental illness. I think every parent does this, anyway. Maybe some have a sense of loss when their teen leaves home. Others grieve over things not turning out how they had imagined – whether in relationships, education, work. But it can be more significant when there are mental health issues, and especially when there is associated alcohol and drug use.

Allow yourself to recognise your grief and your disappointment that some of the things you had dreamed about might not happen – or not in the way, or when, you'd hoped. But then you need to turn your attention back to your child in the here and now. Alongside the challenges they're experiencing, there are still lots of wonderful things. Find and cherish those wonderful things. Sometimes it's difficult, but it's about being in the moment, catching a good moment in between the hard ones – a laugh that you might share in the kitchen, a tiny flicker of the child you know and who is still in there. Find those things, and hold on to hope.

Elliot: It's also true that as a teenager goes through this process of mental illness and recovery, they will change. They won't go back to exactly who they were. This is partly because adolescence is a development stage that involves maturing, and also because mental illness is a life-changing experience. Both they and you will have changed through the experience.

There may be very positive changes where recovery goes well. They may be more independent as they feel more confident in themselves, their identity and their skills to manage their life and emotions. Acknowledge and celebrate those strengths even if they may feel like a distancing from you. They may go out more and need you less. These are positive signs, but I acknowledge they represent a change in the parents' role.

Learn to love and appreciate the changes in your child. Recognise how strong and capable they can be.

- Acknowledge the grieving process that a parent might go through when their child has a mental illness. Some of the things you dreamed about might not happen in the way you'd hoped.
- Take pride in your child's efforts and your role in supporting them towards recovery.
- Catch the good moments in among the hard ones, and find ways to love the child you have.
- Be prepared for your child to change as a result of their experiences – and you will have changed, too.

37.
Sensitive, confident parenting

JK: I have the feeling that parents in New Zealand are not as confident as parents in Italy are. New Zealand parents are a bit more hands-off, whereas Italian parents are not afraid to be dominant. There's an attitude here of 'They've got to find their own way' – which has its pluses – but sometimes kids need a bit more guidance around them.

My dad would call it 'horses for courses'. We're parents. We've got to assess the situation and make a decision about the best way to act. If your child is sick, if they're out of control, you've got to do something. It takes a lot of courage to look after a sick child. But that's when it's time to step up. It's the time to stand by them – and that means listening carefully and taking the load.

Lyndy Matthews (psychiatrist): Sensitive, loving parents fear to intervene too early with this age group because they understand that their child is trying to grow up. They understand that they need to step back and allow the young person their space. And yet this can inhibit necessary action. I would often say to parents in this situation: 'Listen to your gut and go for it, and talk about it with your child and do whatever it takes.'

It's awful to be considered an over-controlling parent, so let's be clear what we mean. I said it earlier: moving in closer to your child because they are ill doesn't mean trampling on your child's rights or telling them what to do. It means working with them collaboratively, and it means *being there*.

Kirsty: Once depression and anxiety have entered the scene, a good deal of parental confidence – or at least the appearance of it – is needed. When depression is severe or if suicidal thoughts and behaviours are involved, it might get to a point where you have to be more proactive than you might normally be with an adolescent, and you might have to say, 'We're getting you some help, regardless of your wishes.' That would be the more extreme end, but it may happen, and as a parent you need to be confident enough to do that.

Elliot: We are aware of lots of examples where adolescents who have been really resistant – even violently resistant – to help have later said, 'I'm so glad now you did that. I know I was awful to you. I know I was angry.'

It's important to see it as the illness resisting help. When people are ill with depression or anxiety, they really are not themselves, and they do sometimes need someone to step in and make decisions for them. The great difficulty in this is that, with adolescents, the natural development is to be stepping back and encouraging them to make their own decisions.

Support for you is vital in this, because it's a really hard call to make. It's not about becoming a helicopter parent – it's about being involved, knowing what is going on for them, so you can make the call when it's obvious that things aren't going right.

Layla (Christie's mum): One thing they tell you is there's no place for guilt. But I do wonder whether if I'd been more involved in Christie's life I would have picked this up earlier, just by being there. As a parent you don't want to think something's wrong; but the lesson I've learnt is: it's OK to think something's wrong with your kid, and to act on that.

We're closer because of what we've been through. We say that, and she says it, too. We've been to the brink of what any parent wants to experience, and we've still loved and accepted her, and she knows that. And we've been angry at her, and she's forgiven us. I want to hold on to that closeness.

So we will consciously stay immersed in her life. We won't be afraid to do that.

Going through this anxiety illness taught me that you have to be the net around your child. They're growing, their brains are still learning to function properly, they're learning to make the right choices – and you need to be there to be able to identify when the right choice is not being made. Everyone needs to make mistakes, but we've learned you need to be involved and engaged and immersed in your kid's life, and there to step in and make a call when you can see something's not right.

- When a child is ill, parents need to move in closer in order to help them.
- It's hard, because in adolescence parents are usually giving their kids more choice and independence.
- Moving in closer doesn't mean ordering them around; it means stepping up and working with them collaboratively. It means being there in order to support and help your child.

38.
What it's like for siblings

Alex (Hannah's sister): I was 13, and my older sister Hannah, who is the person I look up to, one of my main role models, was going through a really hard time with anorexia.

Your sibling turns . . . not into a different person, but they change. It's the illness taking its toll. It was weird to see Hannah not baking and cooking because that's what she loved to do. That was hard. But it's all coming back.

Mum and Dad didn't tell me till I asked them if something was wrong. When they finally told me, they said I wasn't allowed to talk about it to my friends. I'm a very open person, so it was really hard not to. On the day she went into hospital I went to school and broke down. If I had held it in I would have ended up getting sick myself. I kept that a secret from my parents that I'd told my friends, and I was really worried about that as well.

It would have been helpful to have had someone to talk to. It's frustrating. An illness like cancer is talked about all the time. Someone at the same time had a little sister who had cancer, and she stood up in front of the whole class and said, 'This is why I won't be at school so often.' And I didn't have the opportunity to tell a few friends and not feel guilty that I was telling them. It shouldn't be something that you're ashamed of. We've all learnt a lot from this.

In the end I found one or two friends who I could talk to, but then I felt bad because things would happen every day and I thought my friends would get sick of me talking about it. Some of my friends did get sick of me, because I would be upset so often. Then I found I could talk to a teacher who I really liked and trusted and that was really good, and I could talk to them every day.

I've got stronger. I could probably handle situations like that better now. If something happened for someone else, a friend, I would know what it felt like. But I had no one and I was quite young and I was immature. You have to keep a strong mind.

Elliot: When there is a teen in the household with depression or anxiety, a large amount of parental attention and energy is engaged in worrying about and managing that young person. However, depression or anxiety in a family impacts siblings as well. They may feel neglected and frustrated with the amount of parental energy (whether good or bad) that goes into their sibling. They can also feel they are missing out on things, or that the family has changed because adjustments have been made to try and manage their brother or sister's anxiety or depression. Part of this may include a sense of loss through changes in their relationship with their sibling because of the illness.

For a parent, it can be challenging trying to find extra energy for a sibling who is not unwell. However, taking time to do this is essential for them and you. Here are some ways in which to do this.

- Be aware of the impact that depression or anxiety may be having on others in the household.
- Give siblings opportunities to talk about what is going on for them, and to express the mix of emotions they may be experiencing. These might include guilt (*did I cause this?*), anger (*it's not fair!*), anxiety (*will I get it too?*), sadness (*people tease me about it*) or loneliness (*he/she won't talk to me any more*). Be patient, validate their feelings, and help them address these feelings in a non-hurtful way.
- Educate siblings about depression or anxiety, so they can better understand what is going on and why changes may be made temporarily. Don't hide things from them – they will have picked up that something has changed and may piece together information incorrectly. Point them towards age-appropriate information and supports for them, and ways in which they can support their sibling (see the Resources section).

- Help them know what to say if people ask what's going on. Give them age-appropriate brief statements they can use that protect their sibling's privacy but mean they don't have to lie, such as 'They just have some worries at the moment,' or 'It's a bit hard at times, but we're all working together on it.'
- Consider setting them up with someone they can talk with freely and confidentially who knows what is going on and can support them – for example, a school guidance counsellor, a youth group leader, or another adult in the family.
- Ensure they get access to and can be involved with activities and relationships outside the family as well, so life isn't dominated by depression or anxiety.
- Make time for them to have some one-to-one time with parents that is focused just on being with them, and how things are going for them – they still need to talk about their day-to-day worries and goings-on, even if they seem small in comparison to what is going on elsewhere.
- Encourage a relationship with their siblings outside of the depression or anxiety. Make time to do things that strengthen the family and sibling bond. These may initially be very undemanding activities, such as watching a TV programme together or going for a walk. Find ways to have fun together, taking into account the level of energy that will be needed.

Be mindful that siblings may share many risk factors for mental health issues that their unwell brother or sister has. They may be experiencing the stress that can arise in a family where someone is anxious or depressed. Therefore it is important to keep an eye out for signs of depression or anxiety in a sibling, and give them any support they may need.

Mental health can rip through a family, but it can also knit it together. It isn't uncommon for families who come through depression or anxiety to talk about how they are strengthened and closer as a family. Keeping an eye on siblings and their needs throughout the journey is an important part of this.

39.
The journey is hard on parents, too

Mel (Hannah's mum): Being able to separate the illness from the child is really important: 'It's the illness making you say that, and that's not your fault.'

But when you say that the anxiety or the depression or the eating disorder is not the child, that the child is separate from these illnesses, the kid will come back with: 'Why do you say that? It's not separate from me; it *is* me; it is how I'm feeling. Don't say that.' And you can fall into that trap of the kid thinking you don't care about them. It's a fine line between them wanting to be heard and understood, and them feeling negated. And as an untrained parent – *human* – often I felt like, I'm not qualified to be dealing with what feels like such a serious thing. So often I felt that what I said or didn't say was make or break, life and death.

I often didn't remain calm. I think it's important to forgive yourself for not being this paragon of virtue. Who can be? I think that's impossible. A lot of people beat themselves up so badly for things – like, when their kid says 'Fuck you', they say 'Fuck you' back. It's all very well to say that's unhelpful. It's all very well to say, 'Don't feel guilty.' You can't just tell someone not to be guilty or depressed or anxious. You've got to get your head around why you don't need to be guilty. So that for me was part of self-help, really getting my head around the idea that families aren't part of the problem, they're part of the solution.

My mantra was: *The only way out is through*. I love that. We learnt it, too – that the worst moments were necessary. These dreadful moments of your kid being in a foetal position in a corner, and you think, *my functional, normal, happy family has turned into this*. Those moments are awful, but you do come to realise you're going *through* and you're going to come out. This has to happen in order for us to come out the other side.

The other mantra I love comes from FEAST (Families Empowered and Supporting Treatment of Eating Disorders, feast-ed.org): *Feedback not failure*. If something goes wrong – and it will – well, good: that's feedback, not failure. Because we're not perfect and we are learning, and every single case is different.

Catherine (Sean's mum): I've never been angry with him because I just liken it to . . . say he had cancer, I'd never be angry at him for getting that disease. I'd never be angry with him if he was a diabetic. Mental illness is no different. Sure he made some bad choices, but he was an adolescent, and a lot of adolescents make bad choices whether they have depression or not. This was just something that compounded our situation. I felt grief, I felt extreme fatigue, those sorts of things – but I never did feel angry. And Geoff didn't, either.

Elliot: Grief is a complex state that involves many different thoughts, feelings and physical reactions. Parents typically experience it as intense stress. This can include an overwhelming mix of shock, denial, anger (*don't they realise the impact this has had on our home life, work life, relationships?*), anxiety (*will they get better? how safe are they?*), guilt (*did I cause this? should I have noticed earlier?*) and exhaustion. When considerable energy is being expended on the young person, the couple relationship can also suffer, and normal differences in parenting can be exacerbated by the more extreme and challenging behaviours that can accompany depression and anxiety.

For single parents there may be additional stress associated with having less support and fewer resources. For step-parents there may be additional challenges in the context of conflict around their role in parenting the young person through their mental health challenges.

- The stress of journeying with your child through mental illness needs to be acknowledged and addressed by parents and caregivers.

40.
Parent self-care – put on your own oxygen mask first

Elliot: I have a young man I've been seeing for depression. It's a relatively uncomplicated case and he's moving through therapy really well, but it has completely thrown his parents. They are beside themselves with worry, and really struggling to deal with the emotional impact on their lives. They need help – and in fact I have referred them to someone – but it was very difficult for them to acknowledge that they needed help. They felt they should be coping, and strong for their young person.

It makes me think that there needs to be some sanctioning of parents' need for help, because the stress that comes with mental illness is enormous and can challenge parents beyond what they are prepared for. That help could possibly be professional help. You might need help to manage stress – and it's not unusual for parents to develop depression or anxiety themselves in these situations. But it could also be strategic help – taking turns with your partner to give each other time out; or enlisting a friend to be at home so you can go out for a walk. Something that gives you a breather and helps you to cope.

Catherine (Sean's mum): If at all possible, try and get away for some 'couple time'. And while coffees and dinners and movies are a great idea, I'm talking right away from it all – getting some uninterrupted rest for a couple of days! Geoff and I found this invaluable.

And then there's personal self-care, too. I made sure I had the odd massage, manicure, time to read, go for walks – little things. I never lost sight of the importance of making sure I looked after myself.

Kirsty: Some of this comes back to stigma and our reluctance to talk publicly about what we're going through. When we look at the statistics, the studies indicate that about one in five young people will experience mental health issues. That's a few kids in every class – which means those parents will be going through the same thing as you, or will already have gone through it, or will go through it in the future. That's a lot of people impacted by mental illness. And yet we persist in a feeling of shame that stops us talking about it and getting support from one another.

The isolation and shame that parents feel when their child is sick is a huge contributor to stress. Dealing with a situation where an adolescent has depression or anxiety, possibly with attendant behaviours such as truancy, self-harm or substance abuse, means that these times can be almost unbelievably stressful for parents. If they are to help their children, they need to get as much help for themselves as possible – either from friends and family or professionally, or both. You can't do it alone.

Seeking support from others can be challenging, however, as your teen may not want you to tell other family members, and you need to respect this. However you can also discuss with them the importance of support for you, and a safe place (from their perspective) where you can get that. Options might be an agreed family member, other parents, a support group, professionals, cultural or church supports, or even an online anonymous support group.

The great thing about support is it doesn't necessarily need to be someone who knows all the details of what is going on. Support can take multiple forms. It can be someone you talk with about the day-to-day challenges; someone who distracts you, with whom you can do other things that give you a break from the stressors, someone who makes you laugh, someone who gives you courage, someone who supports your wellbeing – for instance, someone you exercise with. The bottom line is that support is necessary. You need to look after yourself so you can look after your young person. Like the airline safety video says, 'Put on your own oxygen mask first.'

Layla (Christie's mum): There was one day when Glen had gone out, and Christie took a whole six-pack of chocolate milk and hurled it at the kitchen wall and it exploded and the chocolate milk went all around the room. I just lost it with her. I gave back what she was giving me. I just wanted her to see what was she doing to us: she was ruining our lives. That was probably the worst moment. Afterwards it felt terrible. But it's human. You have to let yourself be human.

I'd have nights where I'd just cry in bed. Night-times were hard – she'd creep around the house and listen in to us and scream if we were talking about her. Some nights I'd wake up at about 2 a.m. and just sob, and that was my release valve. You have to get the emotion out at some point.

The mental health service gave us homework, too – things we absolutely had to do for ourselves. For Glen it was getting back into his exercise three times a week, and for me it was going for walks. Up to that point we'd found it hard to keep those things going. But I had to do stuff for me and not just be consumed by what was happening for Christie. Whatever you're dealing with as a parent, it's really important to try and keep yourself healthy.

Mel (Hannah's mum): I have been through some really tough times with this, and I was myself really unwell for a while and I became suicidal. I honestly thought they'd be better off without me, because there was so much conflict and so much misery. There were several serious family issues going on simultaneously, and there seemed to be no progress. It was all going backwards. I thought, *OK, this will fix it.* Not so much *this is my fault*, but *this will help*. It wasn't *I can't cope*, but *I think I should go*. I was really depressed. I had a plan – yet I knew that wasn't right, and the only way I could convince myself of that was focusing on how hard it was in families where the parents had died and knowing how hard that was on the kids. I had to *academically* believe that. I didn't really think it applied in my case, but I had to believe it and so I got to a doctor and I got onto an antidepressant. That was part of self-care, getting some medication. Going weekly to a counsellor myself really helped.

My tendency was to drop everything that I usually do; but I did keep playing tennis. While I let some people in on what was happening to me so that I could get their support, I didn't tell others. So it was really neat that my tennis team didn't know. It was business as usual, and a great break.

- When a child becomes unwell, parents can be challenged beyond what they're prepared for.
- Sometimes parents need to seek help themselves. That could be personal support from the extended family or friends, or professional help from a counsellor of their own.
- It's important to take good care of your own physical and mental health. Take time out for you and set up a range of supports.

41.
Advice from the front line

Catherine (Sean's mum): My advice to anyone going through this is: surround yourself with family and friends who are non-judgmental – people who fill your tank. We have been so lucky to have a huge support system. One of our strongest allies has been my mum. Her unrelenting love and support for all of us has been amazing. She has made herself available so many times to be with Sean on his own, taking him out for coffees and brunches – listening to him and offering lots of grandmotherly advice – without being 'preachy'.

Read as much as you can. Google – although sometimes you do get a bit bombarded with so much information. Maybe take a couple of things to work with; don't try and do everything. I discovered information about highly sensitive people (HSP), for instance, which was very helpful. I downloaded a couple of books about HSP and refer to them often. It was like reading about Sean – that highly sensitive nature is often a common denominator in depression.

There's no doubt I've grown through this experience. I've been thinking about how Geoff and I have different ways of going about things when dealing with Sean, but somehow our ways complement each other. I operate on an extremely emotional level – yes, a bit 'mothery'. But I would leave conversations about practical things to Geoff because he's a businessman, a practical thinker, and can see the wood for the trees. I think we worked well as a team. I could cope having Sean in our home for hours on end with him either lying on the sofa asleep, crying, or awake but uncommunicative – I could deal with all that. I'd come in and out of the living room just to be with him, check on him, whatever. Geoff, on the other hand, said that would drive him insane; but he was great with the really serious conversations.

I have never felt shame at any point in our journey. Having depression is nothing to be ashamed of. It is what it is, and you just have to accept it and deal with it, as you would any other illness.

PART SIX
The Unsafe World

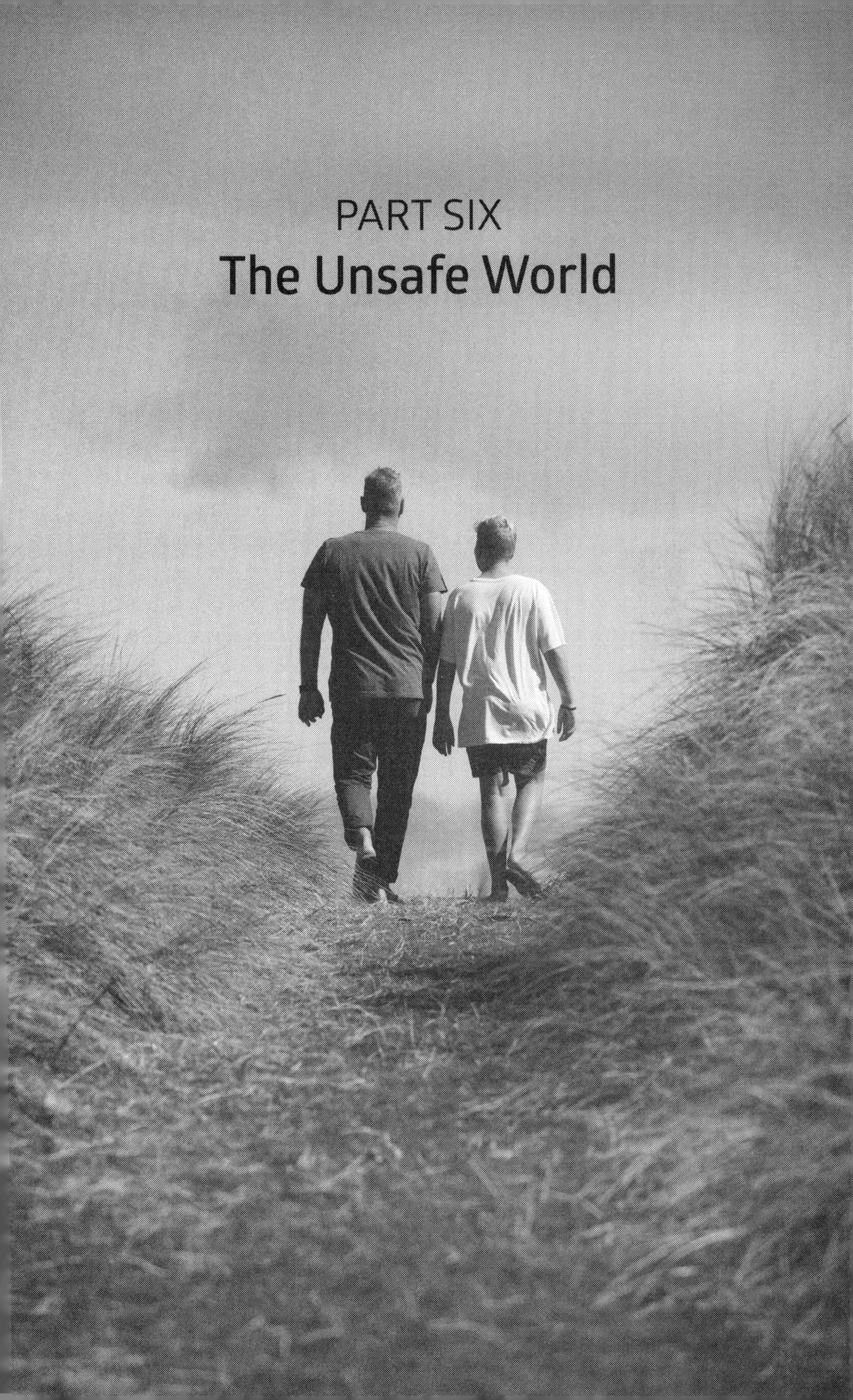

42.
This world we've created

JK: Society is far stronger than us, so maybe we should spend a bit more time trying to change society.

We have a tough culture where people's sensitivities are covered up by a hard shell, and I believe that is one of the things behind the high incidence of mental illness in New Zealand. Look at all the things kids have to deal with. Suicide – we've got one of the highest rates in the world. Self-harm. Bullying – it's a daily fact in our schoolyards. For kids struggling with their sexual identity, there's still plenty of prejudice out there. Social media – where kids think everyone else is happy every day, and there's something wrong with them because they're not.

When you're in depression you don't feel normal. You feel very isolated, that what you're going through is personal. That it's yours. You feel weak, you lose your confidence.

Yet a lot of the things that kids experience are social problems. Kids experience them individually, but they're about the kind of world we live in. Do we want this kind of world? Or do we want a world where problems are shared, and people can talk without fear about what's going on for them?

Once you share something and realise other people are suffering, too, it makes it easier.

43.
Suicide – when it gets so dark

Tomorrow
I woulda spent more time chasing silly dreams
If the world ended tomorrow
I woulda been less focused on the little things
If the world ended tomorrow
I woulda spent more time with my family
Devoted a day to just planting trees
If it all ended, in a splendid type of show
In the morning
I woulda spent more time chasing silly dreams
If the world ended tomorrow
Chorus
When it gets so dark that you can't find your way home
Let your hands reach out to guide you down the road
And when it gets so cold that you can't seem to go on
I'll be there
Said I'll be there
—Pieter T

JK: They talk about suicide being a permanent solution to a short-term problem. My whole motivation is that one suicide is one too many.

Did I consider suicide? Yeah. So I certainly know what that feels like. I can remember driving across the Auckland Harbour Bridge and thinking, *I've had enough, I can't do this any more.*

Did I plan it? No. I was very lucky that I never became truly suicidal. Those thoughts come and go – they pass – and that's advice I give to people.

I've seen the real devastation that suicide always leaves behind it. Mums blaming themselves. Families crippled. It's not the solution.

Jacob: Sometime in the first half of my fourteenth year I tried to kill myself. I was obsessed with getting away from everything. I wanted to go and live in the bush, and I had elaborate plans about how I was going to do that. But I wasn't allowed to go, and there were increasing arguments about it at home. I really thought that if I could do that, everything would be OK.

I was very unoptimistic, very angry, totally trapped inside my own space. I was living inside a grey, heavy cloud. One night I took a lot of something I thought would kill me, but next morning I was still alive. I grabbed the note I'd put outside my door, and jumped back into bed. Mum came up and I told her I was sick, so I stayed home. I was really sick. I couldn't eat anything, I was throwing up and in a lot of pain, although I hid the extent of it. Mum took me to the doctor but of course he didn't know what I'd done, so he just thought it was a tummy bug and said go home to bed. I was home for a week or so. Went back to school.

Then I was called in to the school counsellor and we were talking about how I was doing. 'How are you doing, Jacob?' I must have been talking about how I wasn't feeling that good. It must have been standard procedure to ask if you've had any suicide thoughts. And I was like, 'Yes, I took all this stuff.' She called up my stepdad, John. We went to the hospital, had a blood test. It was shit in the hospital. Didn't want to be there. My liver was damaged, but they said I was lucky and it would recover.

I got referred to the Kari Centre. They wanted to meet with everyone – Mum, John and also Dad. That was not nice having them all in the room together. It was quite hard for the counsellors. Dad's attitude is quite dismissive. He blamed Mum and John for everything – and so I ended up going and staying with him after that.

Dad didn't talk about any of it to me. I remember stealing a few beers and sneaking out into town with a guitar on my back as if that's some kind of . . . like trying to say to yourself that you're, like, free, that it's all OK. Really rotten. Going and sitting down and playing guitar and drinking. On a grassy hill or some shit in the middle of the night. Did that a few times. And then one night I poured some vodka into a bottle and was tiptoeing up the stairs with it and Dad came down, and he was like, 'What have you got there?' He took one sip of it and cast it in my face. We had a violent fight and I ran away back to Mum's. I was very bruised and it was pretty horrible. Didn't see him for a long time.

I thought about suicide a lot around that time. It was a dark, angry, sad time and I put myself in some really dangerous situations.

What held me back was thinking about Mum and my sister and brother. Powerful thoughts. That's pretty much it. What it would do to them. I got to hear all about that when I did it that first time.

Sean: There's all that talk about suicide being selfish and that was a very prominent thing that I'd heard from family members. But when you're going through that you can't really relate. You think it's not selfish.

But when my grandfather died recently I realised what death does to people, and how it reaches the people who are not just right beside you but the people who are beside them and so on and so on. So it doesn't matter how bad you're feeling. It's one person versus a whole lot of people feeling bad. That was my logic when I was feeling terrible. I knew I'd never do anything like that because I love my parents and everyone around me too much, and I realised what it would do to them.

Kirsty: New Zealand has a tragically high incidence of youth suicide: it ranks as one of the highest in developed countries in terms of suicide rates. These are sobering statistics.

Suicide is not a disorder in itself, but is an outcome strongly linked with depression. Postmortem psychiatric studies suggest that 90 percent of young people who committed suicide had a mental disorder at the time of their death; the most common disorder was depression. So depression – particularly severe depression – is a key risk factor for suicide.

Another significant risk factor is a previous suicide attempt. The Canterbury Suicide Project found that of 129 people who had made a serious attempt on their lives, 53.3 percent had made previous attempts. Other significant risk factors include family history of psychiatric disorder or suicidal behaviours; a childhood with adversity or disadvantage; hopelessness; having anxiety or other mental health issues alongside depression; and misuse of alcohol and drugs.

Understandably, there has been much worrying over why so many of our young people kill themselves. Unfortunately, there aren't easy answers, and therefore no easy solutions. Suicide is complex and multifaceted with multiple social and individual contributors. Apart from the risk factors mentioned above, there are social factors that can impact on a young person's risk, such as the economic context and the portrayal of suicide in the media. Researchers are also examining the contribution of other societal factors, such as New Zealand's high rate of alcohol consumption and our 'national stoicism' – where we don't tend to talk about emotional problems and stressors.

Suicide attempts and suicidal ideation (thoughts about suicide) are also unfortunately high among our youth. The Youth'12 Report found that 6 percent of female students and 2 percent of male students had made a suicide attempt during the previous six months; and a startling 21 percent of female students and 10 percent of male students had seriously thought about suicide in the previous 12 months. There is what we call a 'gender paradox' here – it appears that females are more likely to think about and to attempt suicide, and yet figures show that more males die from it. The reasons for this are unclear and complex, but likely contributors may include differences in methods chosen (with males choosing more lethal methods) and differences in help-seeking behaviour and reporting (with females more likely to do this, increasing the opportunities for intervention). Clearly, having thoughts about suicide is not uncommon for our young people.

Given how common it is, how would you know if your young person was thinking about suicide? Firstly, be aware of the risk factors. If they have depression or anxiety their risk goes up. If they have additional risk factors like those mentioned above, it's higher again. Look out for warning signs such as:

- preoccupation with death (through art, reading, music)
- talk of suicide – direct threats, or statements such as 'What's the point in living?'
- changes in behaviour – isolation, involvement in high-risk activities, giving away possessions or sudden appearance of happiness or calm in the context of the above
- mood changes – particularly hopelessness.

As a parent, what can you do about this? It's terrifying to think that your young person may have thoughts of killing themselves. The first and most important thing is: *don't avoid the topic*. There's a myth that if we talk about suicide we will plant the idea in our young person's head. It's apparent from studies like Youth'12, though, that it's not uncommon for young people to already have had thoughts about suicide. Suicide is too prominent a feature of our culture now through media – TV shows, literature and social networks – for our young people not to have come across it already. We're not going to put it in their minds by talking about it – it's already there. The unknown for them is not: *is suicide an option for me?* They already know it is an option. The unknown, the option they aren't so sure about is: *who can I talk to about this? How can I get help?*

This is a hard conversation to have with your young person. There's nothing easy about it. Name that, say to them: 'This is really hard to talk about but it's so important. I'm worried about you. I want you to know I'm here. I can see things are hard for you at the moment and I know sometimes when things are like that people think about suicide or hurting themselves. Have you had any thoughts like that? If ever you find you're thinking about that, come to me and we can talk about it, or I can find you someone for you to talk to.'

You can reference things in the media, TV programmes, the coroner talking about suicide – and use that as a conversation starter. You can talk about it in the third person: ask them if they know anyone who has attempted suicide. Ask them if they would know where to go for help if they were worried about a friend.

The bottom line is that you're saying to them: *I care about you, I'm here. I want to support you in finding options to help you through, and be there in whatever way I can.* You're also saying to them that it's OK and important to talk about this: *you don't keep suicide a secret.*

If you don't think your young person will be honest with you, or you don't feel confident to ask these questions, find someone else they trust to talk with them – such as your GP or a school counsellor or youth leader. I think one of the reasons we get anxious about asking if our young person is having suicidal thoughts is that we don't know what to do if they say yes. It's scary – but it comes back again to sharing the problem: expand the team.

If your child tells you they have had some thoughts of suicide, don't panic. Use the validating approach again. Acknowledge and support their feelings – in particular, how bad they must be feeling to have thought about that as an option. Often what is underlying the thoughts about suicide is not so much a desire to die but a desire for the hurt / shame / awfulness that is their current situation to end. This might be the depression, struggles in a relationship, the endless anxious thoughts – things that can and will pass, even if the young person can't see that right now.

The more frequent and thought-out their suicidal thoughts are – that is, if the thoughts are occurring frequently and the young person has thought about how they might do it – the more serious it is.

Acknowledge how bad things are for them right now. Tell them that there are ways these things can be dealt with; there are ways you can work with them to get through this. They are not alone.

Brainstorm the next step with them – for instance, contacting a GP, school counsellor or youth worker; or, if you're really concerned, call the local mental health team (see the Resources section at the back of the book). Make a plan with the young person about who they might go and see, and when.

Check they are feeling safe in the meantime. If they have any plans to do something and don't feel safe, then they need to see a professional immediately. Otherwise, discuss with them what they might do until the appointment is made. Brainstorm with them things they can do to lift their mood or distract themselves. The Resources section at the back of the book lists a number of sites with suggestions for this.

Let them know that they can come to you at any time – to offload, to distract, to have a hug. Remember you don't have to have, and won't have, the right answers or the perfect thing to say to make them feel better – much as you dearly wish you did. What you are doing here is standing by them, holding the hope for them, and letting them know that they are not alone and they will get through.

Then take the next step with them: take them to speak with the GP or a health professional. Sometimes when you get your young person to the health professional, they might play it down – 'I was just kidding, I only thought of that once and I just said it to rark Mum up' – and the professional might conclude there is no risk and nothing needs to happen. If you are concerned that this isn't the case, you need to collect more information to take back to the professionals. It could be that they just don't have enough information to make a judgment about the risk, so you need to provide them with more details of your concerns and observations. Or it could be that offloading to you, being heard and understood and taking some action has lifted some of the hopelessness and associated suicidal thoughts. Trust your instinct here, and keep asking/checking in.

Whatever the outcome of the assessment is, it needs to include a plan – how to monitor for any ongoing concerns, what to look out for, what is happening to address the things that led to the young person having those thoughts, and where will they/you go if they have these thoughts again – that is, what supports are in place? This is helping the young person see that they have people standing by them.

Levi: Suicide. That was one of those dark, evil things that I used to do, like smashing my head on brick walls.

My dad had killed himself when I was one. I used to have really bad dreams, dreams of *kill yourself because you're worth nothing*. For years

I used to do things because I'd have this dream and I wanted to be with my dad, see who my dad is. I'd try and take my life, but I never could. I've tried a lot.

- Suicide is a permanent solution to a short-term problem, and is tragically common in our youth.
- While the causes of suicide are complex, and likely include societal-level contributions, the strongest risk factors are related to mental illness – particularly having depression or having previously attempted suicide.
- There are warning signs to be alert for: morbid preoccupations, talk of suicide, and behaviour and mood changes.
- It is vital to talk to your young person if you have any concerns for them. Initiate conversations, and convey the importance of them talking openly with someone.
- If your young person does disclose thoughts of suicide, or if you have any inkling of this, link them up with professional help as soon as possible and keep them safe.
- Request input to the professionals working with your young person, and ensure that there is an action plan in place that includes monitoring and response options.

44.
Suicide aftermath

Adrienne (Marly's mum): I was terrified she was going to take her own life. I knew, because I talked to her about it, that she had suicidal thoughts. I could see the blankness in her eyes. I could see her eyes were dead. It was the most terrifying thing. We talked about how to keep her safe. Her father and I are separated and both working, but I got my mother to come and stay to be with her at home. We took it in turns to leave work early and met her off the bus every single day of the week. My ex-partner is a marvellous dad, and he gave up his right to have her at that time so that she could live in just one home for a while.

Some months before, a 16-year-old girl that Marly had been very close to had killed herself. We'd gone to the funeral at school – one of these adolescent funerals. Never again! Absolutely devastated parents and siblings, a shell-shocked school. An outpouring. It showed this spinning photo gallery of this beautiful girl. Happy. What are the children supposed to think? You can be happy – happy then dead? And the power of suicide breaks a taboo. That was what this suicide was like for this population of children. They're so young and so lovely, and they've all got issues and their unhappinesses and all the rest of it, but dead is dead is dead. Whatever fantasy you've got about how life is not worth living, believe me, dead is dead. There was nothing, really, to distinguish this child from any other child. And that's OK as long as you're making some kind of link, some kind of narrative about how she ended up dying. But there was none.

When we got to the auditorium, Marly was shoulder-tapped by the principal to go and sit with the family, because she'd been such a support to the dead girl. And we let it happen. Dear god – I remember Marly's face as she looked at us and did the right thing and went off to be with this family. So she was not surrounded by the strong people who loved her – me and her father and her aunt. She had to go through this entire ceremony trying to comfort the devastated members of this other family. And I feel that was one of the biggest abrogations of parental care that I've ever committed.

Kirsty: Following a suicide, the safest way for communities to respond is in a way that encourages grieving and pays respect to the person who has died, but doesn't sensationalise or romanticise their death in any way.

One of the challenges with New Zealand's small size is that young people can hear about and be exposed to deaths by suicide to such a degree that it begins to become normalised within their peer group. When a young person who has died by suicide is sensationalised in any way through the funeral or media, it can heighten the risk in other vulnerable young people. Facebook and other social media can make this worse with memorial pages glorifying the person who has died and highlighting the peace they will have now. To a vulnerable young person this can be very appealing.

Above all, suicide becomes this option, a feasible option for when things aren't going well, for someone who's in a really high level of distress. If they know someone – or know someone who knows someone – who chose suicide as a method when they were feeling similar distress, it means they are far more likely to consider it themselves. This is what we're noticing around a lot of the youth: that it's become very much an option. Whereas once the thought might have flicked through their head when really low and then been dismissed because it's socially unacceptable or you'd just never do it, now there is that next step that's opened up: *Actually, so-and-so did that and didn't she have an amazing funeral . . . She's lucky, she's not having to put up with this any more . . .* So that next step has been demystified.

My advice for parents is: if you know a young person who has died by suicide, check in with your own kids. 'I heard there was a suicide in the school, in the area. Have you heard anything about that? What are people saying about it? What do you think about that? How has that impacted on you?' Then do the screening mentioned earlier – check with them if they have thought about suicide; check they know where to go or where to take a friend, if they have any such thoughts. Acknowledge the distress the young person must have been under to make such a choice, but also what a tragedy that choice was because it's ended up a 'permanent solution to a temporary problem', no matter how big the problem may have felt at the time. Remind the young person that even if it doesn't feel like it at the time, there are always other choices, and that if ever they feel like that, they can come to you, or go to see someone to get support.

You may get very little back from your young person in this conversation – 'yeah', 'nah', 'no way'. If that's the case, that's fine – you're showing them that suicide isn't a secret and you're happy to talk about it with them and help them get support. If they do say something that's of concern, then you can talk more and walk alongside them to get them the support they need.

- Community responses to suicide need to encourage grieving while avoiding romanticising the young person having taken their life.
- New Zealand's small size, in combination with social media, may increase the potential for suicide to be glorified for vulnerable teens, and so be considered a more viable option for them.
- Parents and caregivers should check in with their teens if they hear about a suicide. A key point to communicate is that while suicide is almost certainly a response to huge distress, it is not – and is never – the only option.
- It is important for parents to check in with their teens following such an event, and to take the appropriate action if they have concerns.
- Even when parents and caregivers don't have concerns, they need to remind their young people where they can seek support if they're experiencing thoughts of harming themselves; and that it's OK to talk about it – any time.

45.
Self-harm

Ellen: My sister is in Year 9, and there's this thing called personal Instagrams and only your really close friends can follow them, and people post things of them cutting themselves and really messed-up things. It's a trend to cut yourself and talk about it. These girls are 13 or 14.

Kirsty: 'Deliberate self-harm' is a term used to describe actions a person can take to deliberately injure themselves, such as cutting, burning and scratching. Among students it is disturbingly common: the Youth'12 Report found that 29 percent of female students and 18 percent of male students had deliberately harmed themselves in the previous 12 months.

Self-harm is different from a suicide attempt, in that the intention is not to die. It can seem an inexplicable and awful thing to do, but self-harm is one way that some young people use to cope with their emotional pain – their really difficult, overwhelming feelings such as sadness, anger or anxiety. Self-harm serves a purpose for the young person. It can be a way to manage their difficult emotions; to give a sense of relief or release; to feel something if they otherwise feel numb or 'not there'; to punish themselves; or a way of asking for help or attention when a young person can't verbalise that.

In some contexts it can also be a way to feel part of a group of young people with similar behaviours. Social media can unfortunately contribute to this, with young people posting pictures of their self-harm, and an element of social pressure comes into play.

Hayley: For maybe a year during Year 10, there was this one girl who went around saying, 'I hope you kill yourself.' She said it to my face every single day. As if I was worthless. She'd walk past and say it quietly, but make sure I heard her. Then she got her friends in on it, and they'd laugh and secretly make fun of me; talk and look at me, then look away and laugh. Fake subtle. They want you to know. It's so obvious that it's directed, but they can say, 'Oh no, that wasn't at you.'

I felt sick with anxiety almost all the time and I trusted no one. By high school, if not before, I was definitely depressed. I was constantly sad and not wanting to be around people, and isolating myself. The anxiety was constant: *does this person really like me?*

I just really hated myself. I self-harmed for a while, cutting myself. That was in the first two years of high school. It made me feel better. It felt like I was killing the thing inside me that made me a bad person; but then the good feeling goes away after a while. It's a really scary thing to do, and the thoughts that are going on in your head are scary. It got so bad that I was like, I wanted to die, basically. Yeah. For a while I thought it would be good to be dead. I wouldn't have to put up with anything. It would be an escape. But after a while I thought, *why should I let them win? Why should I give them the satisfaction?*

Kirsty: While self-harm itself doesn't involve suicidal intent, adolescents who self-harm are at increased risk of suicide. The behaviours can also become difficult for a young person to stop if they don't have other ways of coping with their strong emotions or of asking for help. For some young people the self-harming can also become part of their identity and the social group to which they feel like they belong.

It is important that any young person who is self-harming sees a health professional. It could be that depression or anxiety is an underlying factor, and this needs to be assessed for. Depending on the severity and factors behind the self-harming, counselling is recommended to educate the young person and their families about how to deal with the feelings that lie behind the behaviour, and find alternative ways of coping. The website commonground.org.nz has some useful suggestions about ways to approach your young person, and actions you can take if you are concerned about self-harm.

- Self-harm is an unhelpful strategy used to cope with emotional distress.
- Depression or anxiety can be an underlying factor or source of the distress.
- The young person needs help to deal with the feelings that lie behind the behaviour, and to find more healthy ways of coping with distress. This may require the involvement of health professionals.

46.
Bullying – the living nightmare

JK: Remember that old saying, 'Sticks and stones can break my bones but words will never hurt me?' When I was at school, bullying mostly comprised of people getting physically hurt – you'd get a punch, and if you stood up for yourself you'd get a beating. But I don't think that was nearly as damaging as the kind of vicious stuff that goes on these days. Cutting words are powerful weapons, and I believe they're mostly wielded by insecure, weak people. The person who's bullying is usually insecure, maybe threatened by the accomplishments of the person they're picking on, or their difference. They can make life a living nightmare for the person they're picking on, though.

We're not too good at keeping up with social change. We finally decided, as a society, that physical force wasn't a good thing and we've largely banned it. But we didn't foresee that people would turn to cyberbullying and the kind of verbal playground cruelty that goes on today. Now we need to decide, as a community, what we're going to do about that. It's much harder to police. I suspect it's through people like Nakita and Hayley telling their stories that we'll build a greater awareness and conversation about what's acceptable and what's not.

Also, teachers and caregivers need to pay more attention to what's going on out there for our kids, and shift the outdated thinking that says it's somehow 'soft' to take action against bullying. When it comes to bullying, 'harden up' is causing us all sorts of problems.

Kirsty: The Youth'12 statistics indicate that it is not uncommon for young people to experience bullying: 6 percent reported having been bullied at least once a week, and 12 percent said they had received nasty or threatening messages on their phone in the previous year.

Bullying is not one-off behaviour that occurs between friends when they're upset: it is ongoing, deliberate, harmful behaviours. It can take a number of forms, including verbal (name-calling, mocking), physical (actual or threatened), relational (excluding people from groups, starting rumours), and the more recent development – cyberbullying (threats or unkind comments via text, email or posted on social media).

Ongoing bullying has been linked to low self-esteem, problems at school (including poorer achievement, avoiding and even dropping out of school), depression and thoughts of suicide. It is a serious issue that parents need to be aware of and tackle as early as possible.

Bullying is increasingly seen as part of a complex interaction that can involve the bully, the person being bullied, the social environment, peers and the school and home environments. It therefore often needs a team solution. But the solution can only start once people are aware something is happening. Unfortunately, young people who experience bullying are often hesitant to talk to someone about it. Their self-confidence can be lowered as a result of the bullying; they may feel ashamed and, above all, worried that the bully might retaliate if they find out they've complained. They may also have had a previous bad experience of sharing their concerns and having these played down, dismissed, or acted on in an extreme way that resulted in worse outcomes for them (for example, further bullying by those whom they told on; or their own access to social media removed to stop the bullying).

There are some good online resources and supports for people being bullied and for parents, including cyberbullying.org.nz, commonground.org.nz and kidspot.co.nz.

As a parent or caregiver you can:

- Talk with your young person about bullying, and where they might seek help if this is occurring. Sometimes talking about bullying in the context of someone else can be easier. For example, ask them: 'If you had a friend who was being bullied, what would you do? Do you know someone your friend could talk to?'
- Proactively identify people they would feel comfortable going to if they were being bullied: friends, family, extended family, teachers at school, school health staff or guidance counsellors.
- Sometimes young people don't feel comfortable approaching family or school in the first instance. In New Zealand we are fortunate to have some great phone and online support that a young person can contact, including Kidsline, Youthline, thelowdown and What's Up: see contact details in the Resources section.
- Listen, reassure and don't judge or downplay if your child talks to you about being bullied. Offer them support and comfort, and ask them how it's affecting them.
- Be careful about reacting by jumping in and taking control. This is particularly difficult when you are upset and angry about what your child is experiencing. Allowing them to be part of the solution and active in setting it up will help increase their sense of control and self-confidence again.
- Problem-solve possible options or solutions with them. What these involve will depend on the extent of the bullying and its impact on them. Obviously, the more serious the bullying or its impact, the more immediate and proactive the solution needs to be. Bullying at school will need to involve the school in the solution. All schools will have a policy around bullying, and some will have anti-bullying programmes. Cyberbullying may also involve the school, but there are also a number of immediate solutions to mange the bullying, such as blocking messages and individuals (see cyberbullying.org.nz).

With the One Voice campaign (onevoice.net.nz), Nakita Turner bravely tackles bullying head on and encourages others to add their voice as well. Talk with your young person, have conversations about bullying, encourage them to add their voice and, above all, stand by them.

Jessica: It's all cyberbullying now.
Anish: I got it three weeks ago during exams. Ask fm: it's where people ask you anonymous questions.
Scarlet: Back in Year 10 or 11 people made anonymous websites where they'd put other people's personal or private information to cause drama and get at people, and that caused a lot of distress and upset to anyone caught up in it or involved in it. I remember people getting pulled out of health class because they had to go and see counsellors.

JK: How do you defend against that?

Anish: They can write about you, but you can't do anything about it.
Jessica: You have to think that if somebody is doing it, there's something going on with them as well. But if you're being bullied it's difficult to see it from their perspective, because you're just thinking of yourself.
Scarlet: That website got closed down. I'm not sure how it happened – probably having people being brave enough to speak up.
Claudia (Nakita's mum): If parents have kids who have bullied other kids, they need to help them to own their actions and show them how to put it right. They need to encourage their kid to say sorry and ask for forgiveness. It's about parents being good role models. It's about having character and owning our actions. A lot of kids don't know there's anything wrong with it. They might say, 'It's just a joke', but on the other end their behaviour has caused a lot of hurt. We need to help our kids own their wrongdoings and show them how to have better character.

One Voice

Do they know all the pain that it's causing?
Forcing people to run and hide
With the words that are filled up with poison
And threats that bring us fear
I know that you've had it hard too
But you don't have to go down this way
All your pain can stop if you make a change
One voice can make a difference
One voice can make it right
One voice can change the world
One voice can make it better
One voice can heal the pain
One voice can change the world
—Nakita Turner

Claudia (Nakita's mum): Nakita's journey started when she was six years old. She was very passionate about expressing her feelings through music, and at that young age she stepped on stage for the very first time to perform a song she'd written herself. I watched her, in the course of that one performance, go from smiling and confident, to doubtful, to almost in tears as a group of older kids in the front row mocked her and laughed at her. Afterwards she said she would never play again.

We needed to be the strong voice: We told her, 'That is part of life, but it's not about you, it's about how they were feeling.'

But the bullying continued at school, and she became very concerned with what everyone thought of her. She was changing her persona. We pulled her out of school and home-schooled her for a while, and it was the best thing: she grew very strong in who she was. Then she went back to school, but the bullying continued and there were times she was really down.

In recent years she's become confident about performing again, and she's written her song, 'One Voice', to raise awareness of the terrible bullying that goes on in our schools and our communities.

We'd say to Nakita: 'A lot of kids don't want to be doing what they're doing. We think those kids are craving a good sense of themselves but they've given themselves to the crowd.' This is what the song is about for Nakita: so many people are listening to these negative voices that are pulling them in directions that are not really good for them. We are all individuals, but we have to fit into a mould. When you move away from who you are, that is the darkest place. You want to be able to express yourself freely.

I've always said to my kids: 'Say you're a banana and you're the best banana ever. You look amazing and you taste fantastic, but some people just don't like bananas. You know that some people like apples, so you try and squeeze yourself into the persona of an apple. But someone takes a bite of you and they go, that's an odd-tasting apple.'

In life, we have to be secure in who we are and not be so worried about what others think about us, and listen more to the voices of those who care for us.

We've had to do a lot of work with all our kids on this kind of thing. People have to feed really positive messages to their children, equipping them and strengthening them. Because when you hear about what's going on in the playgrounds, it's wicked.

Now Nakita says that the way she overcame her experiences of being bullied and could move forward was by forgiving the people who have bullied her. *Hurt people hurt people.* So retaliation will never break the cycle. Forgiveness was something that helped her at the time, and it also helps her in retrospect, as she is not carrying bitterness inside her. When people can't let things go, they become bitter.

Something about schools – you have to fight to be heard. Teachers have even said to me: 'Do you think you're taking it too far? Do you think you're oversensitive to the bullying?' I couldn't believe it. This is not taking it too far. Our kids are topping themselves because of this. This is serious.

I think we are all created quite sensitively, but we become harder and harder. 'Toughen up' is the dominant message.

I'd like to see a generation of softness. Embrace sensitivity, because that's where people are open to listen and to care.

Nakita has come out of a dark place. She's seen it and wants to do something about it. She wants to be the voice of the people who were in that place. She wants to start a conversation to say it's not alright. You don't need to go down that road. There's a better way. She knows the bullies are hurting, too, and we need to help those bullies.

Hayley: I never lost my hope that people would wake up and realise that bullying actually really hurts someone. I guess I always see the best in people rather than the worst. Even now, I don't care about what happened then. I don't think about it. If I come across one of the people who were involved I try and be nice to them because they might have things going on. I don't want to be like they were to me. I don't want to be like that to anyone.

But I'm angry – angry that anyone can treat others like that. If I see someone being picked on I think, *that's not OK*. It disgusts me, to be honest. I know what it's like and I don't want to have other people go through that.

Now I think, if I could give advice to a kid going through what I went through, I would say, 'Talk to someone.' I wish I had. Just someone who'll be there and comfort you. Someone you can trust. You can say, 'Hey, I don't want you to act on this situation, but I need to talk to you.'

47. Being gay – from fear to courage

JK: It was only in 1986 that homosexuality ceased being a crime in New Zealand. There have been lots of positive changes over the past 30 years, and lots more social acceptance of gay and transgendered people. But homophobia lingers on, meaning that for some young people it is still terrifying to acknowledge their sexuality.

Elliot: Like Amitai, they know they are gay but they fear social rejection, and rejection by their families. This fear can lead to mental health problems. Young gay men experience mental health problems five times more often than young straight men: they get more depression, anxiety, drug dependence, suicidal thoughts and suicide attempts, according to research published in 2005 by Professor David Fergusson at Otago University's Christchurch School of Medicine.

JK: I'm so awed by Amitai's story. By facing down his fears he's put himself in the generation that will change his community. There's a long way to go, and change takes generations, but it's people like him who make the change. His story takes us from fear to courage, from darkness to light, from sadness to hope.

Amitai: My older sister is lesbian, and after she was confronted about it by my mother she packed her bags and left and never came back. It was years before I saw her again properly. So I used to think *my* only option was to run or die. I remember drinking myself to tears at the prospect of living a life without the love and acceptance of my family, thinking that taking my own life might be a better option for everybody.

I think it was a combination of pressure I felt to do well at university after winning a scholarship to study, alongside trying to adjust to a new city where I knew hardly anyone, that triggered my negative self-talk to start back up again. During the times when it became really difficult to balance my studies, and everything seemed to come at me at once, I started to think, *what is all this for?* I didn't have the busyness of home and family life that could sometimes distract me from reflecting too closely on my life and what was going on. But in this new city I was forced to look at myself and it was scary.

In my moments of complete vulnerability the real culprit of my anxiety and fear would rear its ugly head. I would say to myself, *no matter how hard you try, no matter what you achieve, you will never be able to take away the fact that you are gay and when people realise that, everything you have done will count for nothing.* I thought of all of the young people I had helped lead through school, church and in the community: none of them would respect a faggot, a poof, a homo. I had an incredible amount of self-hate created from how I thought the world would perceive me. Every day was filled with doubt and fear that sooner or later people would know my horrible secret, and in my mind's eye I watched my dreams of ever leading a worthwhile life crash around me. It was overwhelming: *why are you doing this? It's not worth it – just give it up.*

I had entered this dark space before – the pull and drag of hopelessness was familiar to me. A few years earlier I saw death as a sweet release from life; and now in my early adulthood those thoughts of losing control returned and I could feel myself spiralling downwards, darkness creeping over me and seeping into me. I felt frustrated, useless and resigned to the fact there was nothing I could do to get out of this funk after all. This was my life, and my end seemed inevitable.

One day in the street I met a priest I knew well. He seemed to tell I was troubled and he shared a story with me. He told me about his gay cousin who never returned from overseas because he thought he would be disowned by his family. He looked me straight in the eye and said, 'If I could see my cousin again, I'd tell him it didn't matter.' It was so awkward, but at the same time . . . that stuck with me. There were people in my life who I held in high esteem who would not care if I was gay.

I remember bumping into a good friend when I was at uni who I had met at a leadership forum when I was 16. The conversation was so hope-filled and positive. She reminded me of who I was and the leader I was called to be. Later that evening I also bumped into a young Samoan gay couple who I was so shocked to see openly out together enjoying dinner and a few drinks. I realised that actually I might be able to find some happiness like these guys had, and I was more excited about the future.

So for me, recovering from depression has partly been a random sequence of events that prevented me from taking my own life – bumping into people who reminded me of the amazing possibilities my life still had in store for me. I've also clung hard to my Christian faith. I've had to work really hard to believe that's a positive way to live my life, and to separate it out from some aspects of the church community that still engender hate.

Every time I met someone or was in a situation that provided me a glimpse of who I *really* was and the things I could do if I was willing to trust His plan, it felt like it was God talking to me. When I was going through that hard time initially, when I was 15, I felt like I had this epiphany and God – or I can also describe it as a feeling of positive reinforcement – said to me: 'You're sitting down at a door that's closed to you and you can't see the millions of doors that are open to you. And you're crying and weeping at that door. I want you to stand up and choose another door.'

The challenge of learning to love yourself isn't unique to people struggling with their sexuality. I think people are constantly trying to accept themselves and sit comfortably with their human nature. We're also searching for somewhere to belong and to be loved. And I'm learning that it doesn't actually matter if that involves a lot of people or just one – the fact that love exists and is possible is something invaluable to building your resilience and keeping you well.

Elliot: As JK notes, society has made some big steps in accepting more diversity around sexuality. However, at an individual level, for many parents hearing that your child is gay can be extremely overwhelming or distressing. It can be experienced almost as a grief reaction, with a sense of loss around what was expected and hoped for. Even where the parent is comfortable with homosexuality, they may still worry about their teen going through life subject to prejudice simply for being gay. As is painfully clear from Amitai's story, it can be hugely challenging for a young person to come out/reveal their sexuality to their parents and family. What needs to be kept in mind is that while disclosing one's sexuality can be a very challenging and painful process for all concerned, not doing so may lead to much more distress in the long term for that young person. It is absolutely vital that even when parents may not be accepting of more diverse sexualities, they communicate through their words and actions that they love their child regardless of their sexual orientation. They need to be mindful that their teen is trying to be honest with them about their sexuality and developing identity. It can be difficult for both the young person and the parents to navigate the changing views around sex, gender and sexuality. There are organisations such as Rainbow Youth (see the Resources section) that can help parents come to terms with their child disclosing that they are gay. Commonground.org.nz also has some great suggestions on how to have supportive conversations around this topic. Other options for parents include talking to others who have gone through this, or seeing a therapist who has expertise in the areas of sexual identity and orientation.

- Consistent with being part of a minority group that is often marginalised, gay teens are at a higher risk of experiencing mental health difficulties.
- Disclosing being gay can be a very challenging and painful process for both teens and their parents.
- It is important to love your child regardless of their sexual orientation.
- Support in coming to terms with having a gay child can be found from organisations, people who have been through the experience themselves, and from specialist therapists or counsellors.

48.
Social media – happy, shiny people

Sophie: Instagram: it all looks so good.
Lou: They only post the good aspects of their life. Not everyone has those lives, but being able to decipher through is hard.

Kirsty: Social media has become an incredibly important part of young people's lives, and one that is not well understood by many adults. Of course, there are dangers inherent in sites such as Facebook, Instagram and so on – the dangers of hyperreality; the dangers of anonymous bullying – but they do play a role in allowing young people to explore their sense of identity and find support.

JK: There's got to be a limit, though. I put my foot down when Luca was getting on Facebook first thing in the morning.

For me, social media is about having control of it, not it controlling you. I don't need social media to connect with people. If you've got someone on your Facebook page but you won't cross the street to say hello to them, you should take them off your Facebook page.

I use Instagram because my kids, cousins, nieces and nephews are all on it. But I choose who follows me. I don't want any more friends than I've got, and I don't want random people knowing who I am or what I do. People say to me, 'Why can't I follow you?' And it's easy for me to say, 'It's just for my immediate family.' For me, it's very personalised around the lives of my kids.

In general, I think that social media doesn't promote courage.

It's much harder to say something to someone's face than it is through media, and that scares me. As for kids dumping each other by text: gutless. Bullying over social media is a real problem, and the kids who are doing it don't seem to have any sense that what they're doing is real.

Matt (Levi's new dad): It's hard to talk about mental health issues without acknowledging the kind of society we live in. Everything around us, the ads on TV, even on Facebook with our friends – they're not real; they're hyperrealities.

There's this expectation that, *if I only get there, I'll be happy*. I think the reality is that happiness as it looks on TV and Facebook is an illusion. It's not actually real. Yet because of the images we're bombarded with, we don't think it's OK to be sad. People with depression have a double burden because as well as feeling so sad, they feel that they are not living up to the expectations of what happiness is.

We're all guilty. You have a good night and you put it up on Facebook and it just looks awesome – but the photos never tell the full story. The realities aren't displayed. Last week at the youth centre I work in, I saw a girl on the computer and I watched her whole demeanour change from something she was looking at – she slumped down. I asked her what had happened, and she said, 'Oh, they went out and I wasn't invited and it looks like they had an awesome time.' She was hurting, and it probably wasn't even real.

Alex (Hannah's sister): A lot of girls and boys look up to cover girls on magazines. I've seen a little clip about what they actually do to photos in Photoshop – they change everything. It makes me so angry. The other day I came across this page, a website that sold underwear, but none of the models had been Photoshopped, and it made me happy, because that girl when she sits down, she does have rolls on her stomach; whereas when you see, especially on those kids' mags like *Seventeen* or *Girlfriend*, they've always got these people with perfect faces, perfect features, and you think, *oh I don't look like that*, and you end up doing stuff and it gets you into bad places.

Brook (youth worker): If you look at the social media world and the mass media world, everything is great. Lorde's just sold a million albums in the US. Look at the new feed on Facebook and Instagram: everyone's having such a wonderful time. *Not me.* So have we actually been good as a society at teaching adolescents how to live in the natural low?

Layla (Christie's mum): Through this experience we've gained a really good understanding of the perils of mobile phone contact, and I've encouraged Christie to really limit her use of the mobile phone to confirm appointments. Christie was desperate for social contact, so when a friend said, 'I might come over and see you', in her mind someone was coming over to see her. But then two hours later they'd go, 'Soz, can't make it now', and she'd crash because it was such a letdown.

But if you talk to a person on the phone you can sense the situation better – whether they're disappointed that they can't come, whether it's because mum or dad aren't around and they can't get there, or whatever. So we've said to her that if she's making arrangements she needs to talk to them on the phone.

Text conversations are not tangible – it's too easy for them just to go, 'Oh, soz . . .' as if nothing matters. You don't know the state of mind of someone who's receiving your text, as innocent as it may seem. We need to teach our kids that good, healthy communication does involve a degree of thought and consideration for the recipient. The remote communication of texting takes it away completely.

Kirsty: Social media and the internet aren't all good or all bad. They can be either, depending on how they are used.

Some good things about social media and the internet in relation to mental health include:

- increased access to information
- increased access to supports
- access to broader social supports and groups (this can be an advantage in particular for minority groups).

Potential pitfalls can include:

- exposure to cyberbullying
- exposure to sexual solicitation
- easy access to inappropriate information (for example, how to commit suicide)
- addiction to social media
- distortion of world view and associated negative impact on self-esteem.

When children are young, parents can exert some control over internet use at home. However, adolescents can increasingly access the internet out of the home on a smartphone, and thus they need to learn how to self-monitor. Management of the internet and social media to minimise any impact on mental health will ideally become an ongoing discussion between the young person and the parent. Some tips for understanding and managing the impact of social media on your young person include the following.

- Get involved early. When they first start using social media they don't mind being your 'friend', and this provides opportunities for monitoring, discussion and learning how to manage the potential risks. Find out about what sites or apps they use and the potential strengths and pitfalls of these. Have conversations with them about this, including how they will manage any pitfalls.
- Talk with them about the pros and cons around social media: how it's useful, what they've seen that isn't useful (for instance, cyberbullying, inappropriate material, things that made them sad, mad, jealous), and how they've dealt with it.
- Talk about the difficulties of taking something back once it's been posted – both words and pictures – and how even apps that delete the message soon after reading can have a screenshot taken and forwarded on. Talk about the implications of the online footprint they are leaving (for example, a future boss or partner might see it).

- Ask them what they are learning at school about social media. Our son's school teacher gave the class a great lesson on one of the negative aspects of social media when he talked to them about how they could have 500 friends on Facebook, and on any one day one of them might post a picture of themselves doing something fun. Their Facebook feed then becomes full of all these other people having lots of fun, and it can warp their view of what life is really like. What it doesn't show is the 499 other people carrying on life with its normal ups and downs, or the 10 other photos taken at that time where that person didn't look happy or beautiful – that they didn't post.
- If you come across something on their social media sites or hear about something that concerns you, don't overreact. Use it as an opportunity for discussion. Remember that young people display their lives through social media. Think back to what you may have said in conversations with friends when upset or angry; now it's just online for more people to see.
- If you are worried about your teen and don't have access to their social media, ask someone who does, such as a sibling or older friend, to keep an eye out for you.
- Encourage your teen to be aware of the impact of their social media use on their mood: do they feel better or worse after using it?
- Encourage them to be active and discriminating – for example, being mindful in their decisions about who to have as friends; deleting posts or pages that impact negatively on them; and not engaging in cyber arguments.
- Encourage them towards the good uses of media: connecting with other family and friends who can be mentors and supports for them; or connecting with websites/Facebook pages/Twitter networks that support healthy lifestyles, and with likeminded people.
- Encourage them to have an active life outside of social media, and to have periods during the day, week and year that are 'technology-free'. Turn Wi-Fi off at a set time at night, and

leave phones, computers, etc. in the lounge to restrict night-time access. NB: you will need to model this as well!
- Point them towards websites such as netsafe (netsafe.org.nz) that have good resources on the internet and cyberbullying.

In her book, *Sex, Drugs 'n Facebook: A parents' toolkit for promoting healthy internet use*, Dr Megan Moreno outlines a useful model for helping young people develop healthy internet habits. It includes:

Balance – Encourage keeping a healthy balance between online life and offline life. Address the issues of time spent online (how much and when); potential overreliance on the internet for social life; and the emotional impact online experiences can have.

Boundaries – Develop boundaries by discussing key topics. These include what information (including photos) it is appropriate to post publicly and to share with others; the concept of 'privacy'; what 'friends' they have online; and whether one's values or moral boundaries should be different online versus offline.

Communication – Establish good, ongoing communication to assist with setting up and maintaining good balance and good boundaries. Like all good communication this involves actively listening, understanding your young person's world, problem-solving, and not overreacting or lecturing!

If your young person is suffering from depression or anxiety, be aware of any role social media might play in this. Is their mood better or worse after their social media use? Is it tapping into their strengths and building resilience, or does it feed into their depressive or anxious thinking? Encourage your young person to think about these questions themselves, and the balance and boundaries they have online.

- Find out about social media and the internet yourself.
- Have ongoing conversations (not lectures!) with your kids about the pros and cons of social media and the internet.
- Encourage balance and boundaries in their use of social media and their online presence.

49.
Getting out of it

Jim: I was going to a soccer game with my dad and he said, 'If you're ever thinking about smoking just come to me and we'll smoke a packet of cigarettes together.' I've never smoked. Maybe if Dad had said, 'Don't smoke or do drugs,' I might have tried it.

Sophie: If your parents are interrogating you, you might do the things they said not to do.

Flora: Teach us the risks: 'Maybe a couple of drinks is OK, but drink responsibly.'

Jim: And don't keep pressuring us every five seconds.

Lou: Trust your kids until you have a reason not to.

Flora: When we were doing health we learned that one of the protective factors is setting boundaries. You need it to a degree.

Sophie: Yeah, like: 'We know you're going out to drink, but don't come back wasted.' My parents take everything very seriously, but my mum will kind of do it in a joking way which makes it much more comfortable. She finds out what she wants, but it's not a pressure thing and I don't get into trouble.

Karl: Parents should show that they care about what's going on in your life, what you're doing and the decisions you're making.

Ellen: They should show an interest in your everyday life, not just when you're in trouble.

JK: It's really hard for anyone in this country to tell their kids not to drink or binge drink because society says it's OK. It's totally normalised and accepted. It's a tragedy.

I love New Zealand. I think that as a nation we have heaps of strengths. We have a real we-can-do-anything attitude – have a go, no fear! We're hard workers. You want to get something done, you get a Kiwi: there are Kiwis all around the world getting things done. So there are lots of positives; but we've got a few things to work on. Basically, I think if you took the alcohol out of the equation, we'd have a pretty perfect society.

There is a series of ads on TV telling people not to drink and fry – pissed young people saying, 'Don't go home and cook.' Those ads annoy me a lot. The way I see it, we're sanctioning people to drink till they can't cook properly. Pissed people on TV giving a safety message? That's ridiculous. The problem is not the cooking – the problem is that our youth are getting absolutely pissed every Saturday night, and as a society we just laugh at it and say, 'Don't cook.' They're not drinking to moderation.

To me, the problem is our binge-drinking culture. The problem is, you're so drunk you can hardly stand up. We've all done it – but that way of drinking is behind kids getting killed on the roads, teenage pregnancy, unwanted sex that just makes kids feel really bad about themselves. And there's a lot of evidence that our high use of alcohol and drugs has consequences for mental health as well.

Jacob: Even now, I'm not sure exactly about the relationship between my drug-taking and my depression, but it was easier for people to relate to me as a person with drug problems than a person with depression – and that was right through the system, from school, to rehab and even at home. Even when I was only 14 or 15. But I think there's a wider problem, that as a community we don't really know how to look after those who are mentally ill.

I can't say if the weed supplemented my depression thoughts that were already there, or if it's the other way round. I think it's a bit of both. My state of mind at the time was very unoptimistic. I was incredibly angry at everything. I felt very angry at the world and the people around me and I felt very obsessed with that.

JK: When I was mentally ill I used alcohol as a relaxant. You kid yourself it's helping, but you just feel even worse in the morning.

I tell my kids the truth. I say, 'We've got a binge-drinking problem in this country, and you need to be able to say no and not be peer-pressured into drinking, and you probably won't have a lot of friends.'

I've always said that the strength of your parenting is in what happens when you're not there. But you can never underestimate the societal pressures our kids are under.

JK: Do you think alcohol is a cultural tradition in New Zealand?

Adam: Yes.

Kirsty: Is there much pressure at school to drink to be part of the in group?

Scarlet: I think there is.
Adam: Especially at the beginning. I didn't for ages; because of my sport, I took pride in not drinking. But I got stick for it.

Elliot: Adolescents with depression or anxiety will often drink to make themselves feel better – to dull their feelings, and to get those brief 'ups' that alcohol can provide. The danger is that substance abuse can become a problem in its own right, in which case they may need specialist help to deal with it. But if it hasn't got to that stage, then treating the depression or anxiety will often quite naturally cause the substance abuse to remit.

The picture isn't good. The New Zealand Mental Health Survey found that over a third of young New Zealanders aged 18 to 21 are at risk of alcohol-related problems each year because of their binge drinking and/or hazardous drinking: 'The onset of substance use disorder occurs mostly in the late teenage years and early 20s with 75 percent of those who develop substance use disorder doing so by 25 years of age' (p. 140). It also found that people with substance use disorders often experience other disorders such as anxiety or depression.

The Youth'12 Report on secondary-school students painted a similar picture: 57 percent of students had tried alcohol, 45 percent continued to use it, 18 percent drank weekly or more often, and 23 percent had engaged in binge-drinking (five or more alcoholic drinks within four hours) in the past four weeks.

Along with alcohol, New Zealand adolescents are significant users of cannabis. Both the Christchurch and Dunedin longitudinal studies found that by age 21 nearly 80 percent of young people had used it on at least one occasion, and 10 percent had become heavy users 'consistent with a diagnosis of cannabis dependence'. Heavy cannabis use was more common in males and among Maori (Gluckman Report, p. 257).

So there's definitely a problem – and the consequences are serious. Alcohol affects the chemistry of the brain, increasing the risk of depression. And mental disorders such as depression, anxiety and suicidal thoughts are more common among adolescents who are heavy cannabis users.

Jacob: I was expelled from my high school at the end of my fourteenth year, but they said I could get back into school if I went to a rehab centre, the day programme. I thought it was the end of the world. I was there for about six months. I don't know what I think about that place in retrospect. You're put with people who take far worse drugs than you do. I was only 15 with marijuana and depression problems, pretty destructive towards myself.

I'm not sure I had a thought at any time that I truly wanted to give it up. I probably really wanted to feel much less depressed and all, but . . . I can now relate depression, my mental health, to my drug use, but I couldn't back then, even then, after that. I did get back into school, but failed a drugs test and was about to be expelled again.

So Mum got me into an alternative school. There I began smoking heaps – several times a day, every day; and at last I started recognising it as something that I wished I could stop. I was realising how unnormal that is, and not cool – and not being able to stop.

I'd stopped seeing my mates, partly because I was smoking a lot more. I couldn't cope, I wasn't social, I couldn't be around people. It made me paranoid and anxious.

I'd smoke and think about how I wanted to stop. That school promoted this whole 'do what you want' idea, and that fitted perfectly with me. It was probably really great for people who aren't really fucked up.

I left school with no qualifications. I started a course at tech, and I finally got kicked out of home. I got a flat and smoked a lot of weed – I'd go for days without eating because I'd spent all my money on weed. Yet somehow things weren't so dark any more. I was still depressed but not suicidal.

And then I came home and had a little play at pulling myself together. I figured I was going to fail my course, so I stopped smoking weed and I worked hard and got good feedback, and that felt really good. I had some good experiences and got a job. Then I started smoking weed again, but by this stage I knew it wasn't helping me. It brought back my feelings of depression.

Sean: I was drinking a lot at the time. That led to a couple of crashes in my car where I just fell asleep at the wheel. I've had two convictions and that's lucky, considering. I don't know what I was thinking, now that I look back. That was stupid. I was doing it every night – mixing my meds with alcohol.

Prescription medication was a big thing for me. I got hooked on anti-anxiety pills: I was prescribed a massive dose over several months, and although my parents felt it shouldn't be prescribed like that, it suited me not to question the dose. I was abusing it, mixing it with alcohol.

I've cut back a lot on my drinking since then. Pretty much my last DUI was the big eye-opener, and because of my convictions I went up to CADS [Community Alcohol and Drug Service]. I've been there and done two Bridge programmes [an alcohol and drug treatment programme run by the Salvation Army] and it's been interesting – and being able to talk to other people about the same experiences, all aimed at alcohol abuse and drug abuse.

I think smoking marijuana probably contributed to my staying depressed; I know it didn't help. But it's a strange thing when you're in that mindset. You can't tell yourself that it's not going to help because instantly it does. It's hard to care about the long run when you don't really care about tomorrow.

I just always felt I needed something. It's weird. I guess you could think of it as a numbness. I don't any more. I'm not using it like I was.

Elliot: Clearly, there are major issues for us as a society here. The Gluckman Report was frank in its assertion that we need to find 'constructive ways and means of regulating the use of alcohol by young people and mitigating the adverse effects of alcohol misuse is a matter of high priority in the area of adolescent policy' (Gluckman Report, p. 238).

It is not uncommon for people who experience anxiety and depression to also have problems with substance misuse. One reason for this is that substances can be used as a source of temporary relief from anxiety or depression, despite the long-term harm this can cause. This is sometimes referred to as 'self-medicating'.

Parents often feel that their young person's alcohol use is out of their control as they become more independent and peer-influenced. This isn't the case. Parents' attitudes and what they communicate to their children about alcohol remain an important influence. Have conversations about drug and alcohol use with your children using natural conversation starters – seeing people who are drunk on TV, reading things in the paper, querying what they have seen in their friends or others when they have been out. Be open with them about why some people use substances, and the impact it can have on their mental health.

Model appropriate alcohol and drug use: your kids will likely learn more from what they see you doing than what they hear you saying! Young people's choice in using alcohol or drugs to manage their mental health will be influenced in part by what they have observed around them. As parents, think about how you use alcohol and drugs socially, and how you model ways of coping with stress and distress. Help your young person identify and find ways to manage stress and distress that don't involve alcohol and drug use, and ways to interact socially that don't revolve around alcohol. Brainstorm with them strategies to use when they feel under pressure socially – a set text message they can send you to signal they need to be picked up; statements they can use as an out, such as 'No thanks, mate, I've got sports tomorrow, we need to win.'

If you are concerned about alcohol use, watch for the warning signs (see over), and be aware of how much your young person is drinking. According to Youth'12, the most common source of alcohol among high-school-age drinkers was parents (60 percent). Therefore, thinking about any role you may play in their alcohol use, and forming strong relationships with clear lines of communication with your child's friends' parents, will be important.

Alcohol.org.nz and drugfree.org note the following as possible warning signs your young person is misusing drugs or alcohol.

- repeated health complaints such as vomiting
- changes in sleeping patterns
- mood changes, especially irritability
- starting arguments, withdrawing from the family or breaking family rules
- falling grades, failing exams, missing assignments, frequent school absences or discipline problems at school
- changes in social activities and social groups or friends
- coming home drunk
- clothes, breath, skin, etc. smelling of alcohol (or increased use of mints or gum to cover breath, or scents to cover smells in rooms or on clothes)
- missing sport, school, family events
- secretive or deceitful behaviour (for example, making constant excuses, avoiding eye contact)
- alcohol, money or valuables going missing from home
- drop in appearance or hygiene
- changes in behaviour (for example, not being where they said they were going to be)

A number of these obviously cross over with adolescence and symptoms of depression, so context, the number of signs and your gut instinct all need to be taken into account. You can't go wrong in having a conversation with your young person. Drugfree.org and commonground.org.nz have suggestions and videos about how to have these conversations with your young person. Be aware, when you're having such conversations, of the reasons why your young person may be misusing drugs and alcohol – social pressures, symptom management, coping strategies and addiction may all play a part. To deal with the alcohol and drug use, the contributing factors need to be identified and dealt with.

There are a variety of options if a parent is concerned about their young person, depending on the seriousness of the problem and the underlying issues. A good place to start is alcohol.org.nz: it has a helpline and useful resources for parents concerned about their young people, and it gives advice and details regarding possible service options in your area. If the alcohol and drug use is symptom management for underlying depression or anxiety, it needs to be addressed in the context of treatment for these. If the substance use is not related to anxiety or depression, specialty alcohol and drug services may need to be involved.

- Alcohol affects the chemistry of the brain, increasing the risk of depression.
- Mental disorders, such as depression, anxiety and suicidal thoughts, are more common among adolescents who are heavy cannabis users.
- Have conversations with your kids about alcohol use and misuse, and model appropriate use.
- To deal effectively with alcohol and drug use, the contributing factors need to be identified and addressed.

50.
Eating disorders

Elliot: A number of the young people we interviewed for this book developed an eating disorder in the context of untreated anxiety; and depression was frequently also part of the picture. Eating disorders are serious, and they are the mental health diagnosis with the highest death rate; so if you have any concerns that your young person may have an eating disorder, seek help immediately.

Layla (Christie's mum): Christie developed anorexia when she was 12. Looking back, there was a perfect storm of contributing factors.

Anorexia is an expression of an underlying anxiety, I believe. For Christie, it was centred on friends and fitting in. We had seen her as far more resilient than she was, far more carefree than she was. But she had these anxieties that are really human anxieties: *do people like me, do I fit in, do they want to be my friend or are they just being kind?*

There are also personality issues. Christie is highly competitive and has a lot of self-discipline, and that's what it takes to stop yourself eating, obviously. We know now that puberty can be a trigger; plus, a lifelong friend of hers moved off with another group of friends.

Suddenly Christie was a bit lost. She couldn't quite place herself.

She hooked up with a group of girls who started complimenting her on how slim she was, and it seems that just triggered something in her mind: approval. It wouldn't have been a conscious decision.

I noticed little things. It started with a desire to make her own lunch, and I thought, *great!* Then I noticed she was cutting back on portions. One day I was checking the lunch she had packed and I saw that she had taken only about three spoonfuls of pasta from the night before. So I filled up her lunchbox and put it back in her bag. She felt it was heavier, opened it and went ballistic. She hurled her lunchbox across the room, completely out of control. I said, 'Christie, why does that matter?' and she said, 'Because now I don't know how much I'm eating.' That's when I thought, *we've got a problem here*.

I immediately made contact with a psychotherapist who specialises in eating disorders and she told us about family-based therapy (FBT), an approach that's having great results internationally. The latest studies, by the University of Chicago and Stanford University in the United States, show that by the end of 6–12 months of the treatment plan, about 80 percent of patients are weight-restored and their periods have started again. Indeed, less than 12 months on, Christie has now reached 95 percent of her goal weight and is well in terms of having normal responses and reactions to food. FBT doesn't focus on the causes of the illness – it's all about eating, getting well. You as the parents take control of the eating. There's no 'We would like you to . . .'; there's just 'You eat that and you eat it now and you do not move until you've eaten that food' – which may well come hurling back at you across the room. It's hard, but it works.

'As parents,' the psychotherapist said, 'I want you to think about the thing that would make you most anxious. And then imagine I say to you, "You've got to do that thing now." How would you react?'

I've got a terrible fear of heights so I said, 'If you took me up the Sky Tower and made me walk around the outside edge I would be a blithering mess.'

'Well,' she said, 'take that and magnify it by 100 and that's what Christie is dealing with.' That really helped, because it made me realise early on how afraid Christie was.

The psychotherapist also said, 'Christie's not chosen to get this illness – and it is an illness, no different to her getting glandular fever.' That really helped, too, because suddenly every behaviour that came back at us – the screaming, the physical lashing out – we could say, 'She's not choosing to do this.'

The psychotherapist also said that Christie's dad Glen and I had to work as a team. 'You've got to be the net that encloses your daughter and you're not going to let the anorexia get through. So imagine you're a net and you're shielding Christie and you're keeping the anorexia back.'

A lot of anxiety treatment is about gradually confronting the fear. If you're afraid of spiders, the treatment will be the spider over there, closer, closer, and eventually you'll hold the spider. But with eating disorders you don't have the luxury of time, because that patient will die if they don't eat. It's the mental illness that results in the highest number of deaths, either through starvation or complications associated with that. Heart failure is a very real risk. It's a very misunderstood disease. For me, putting it in the camp of anxiety made it much easier to deal with.

I really hated the thought that people might label Christie as being vain, or 'one of those silly girls who just won't eat'. I myself had probably thought that in the past, but actually it's far more complex. It might start with a desire to lose weight, but then it takes hold and becomes bigger than that.

Elliot: FBT, which is also referred to as the Maudsley model of family therapy, or the Maudsley approach, has a strong evidence base for treating anorexia nervosa in adolescents. Other treatments have not been researched sufficiently with adolescents to qualify as established evidence-based interventions. Research is ongoing into approaches such as cognitive behaviour therapy and interpersonal therapy, which have been shown to be effective in treating bulimia nervosa in adults. The treatment of eating disorders is complex and specialised, and this is reflected in the development of multidisciplinary specialty eating disorder services in New Zealand. Websites with further information on eating disorders are noted in the Resources section.

- Eating disorders such as anorexia and bulimia nervosa are mental illnesses that include symptoms of anxiety and may be accompanied by depression.
- Because of the serious physical health complications that can occur with eating disorders, it is important to seek specialist professional support if you have concerns about your teen in this area.

51.
Swimming against the tide

JK: Mental illness continues to grow, so there must be something about the way we've constructed our lives that is contributing. It strikes me that there's a contradiction between social pressure and what it takes to be well.

Elliot points to the ideas of positive psychology, such as *be grateful* or *do things for other people.* Ideas like that are quite radical because they're against the way society pushes us. With the 'I' society that we live in, people think, *I won't do something for someone else, I'll just do it for me.*

For mental wellness, you probably need to behave a little bit differently from how society is telling you to behave. Society is saying *go fast*; mental health is saying *slow down, savour the moment.* Society says *every man for himself*; mental health says *when we take the time to be kind to others we not only make a better world, but we feed our own happiness as well.*

Hayley: I was shocked by all the backstabbing that went on between the girls at high school. I don't know at that point if it was particularly aimed at me; I think it might have been the culture. Maybe by that stage I was very sensitive to it. They would say things like: 'You're ugly!' or 'You're a bitch.' It's mostly girls who talk about other girls. They do it secretly behind backs. If they don't like one person, they'll have a massive gossip session.

Claudia (Nakita's mum): In our culture, quite often we laugh and mock – we need someone to say that what we're doing is not very nice. It needs to come from families: everything has to start within your own family ethos. A lot of parents don't realise their kids mimic them, using put-down language. These are attitudes that will be passed down from generation to generation.

Parenting classes can help parents to break the cycle.

Nakita wrote a song about her little sister who had spina bifida, called 'You Will Be Loved', and after it was played on the *Sunday* programme on TV she got so many letters from people saying, 'Because you were so vulnerable and shared your feelings, I can face my feelings.'

PART SEVEN

Resilience

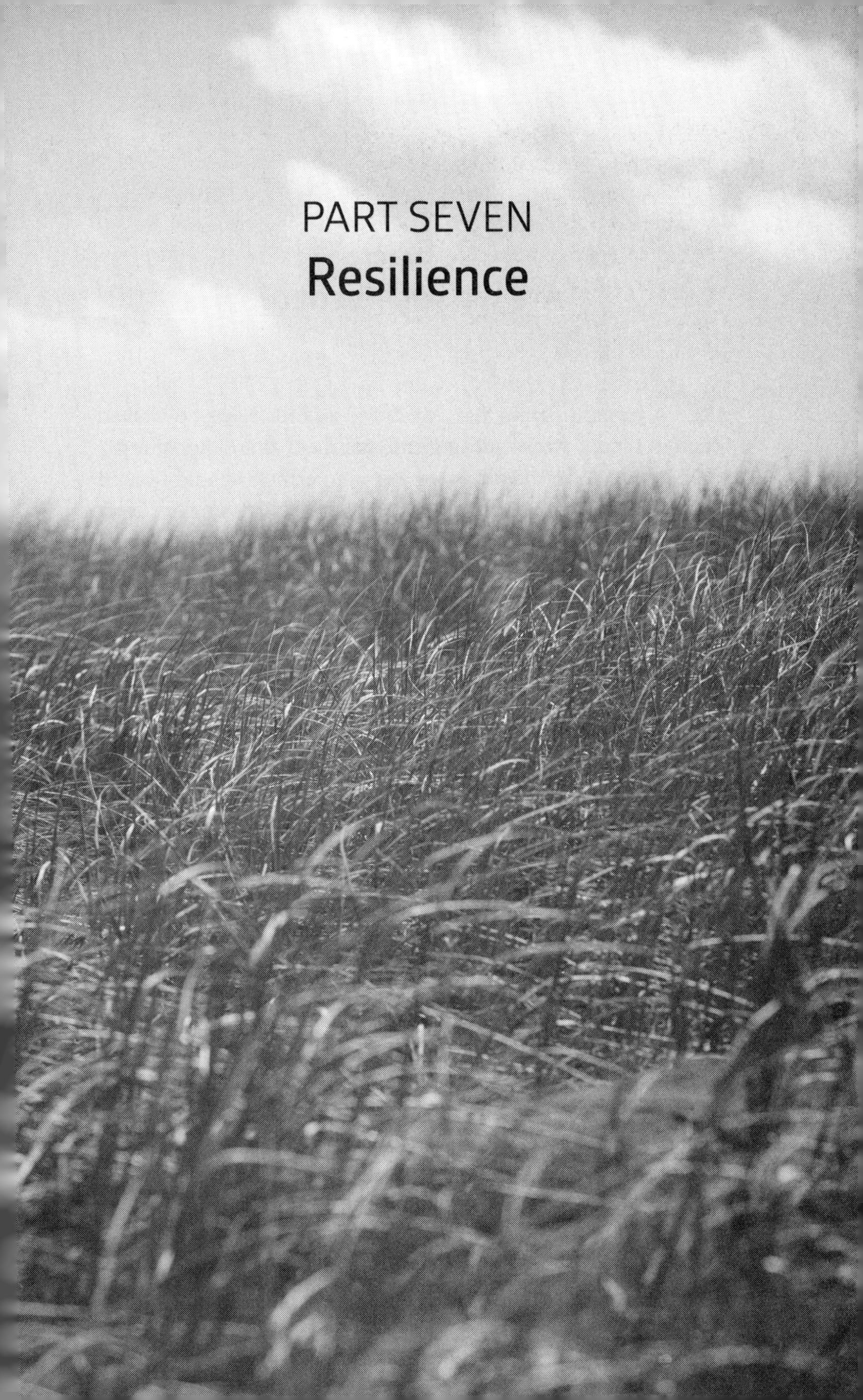

52.
Are we still needed?

JK: A friend of mine has two boys, and for years he walked them to school every morning and met them after school for the walk home. Then the older boy began intermediate and wanted to walk by himself, but my friend still walked his younger son to primary school. Then came the day when the older boy began high school, and at the same time the younger boy began intermediate. Now, neither wanted their dad walking them to school any more. 'I'm not needed any more,' my friend said. He was partly joking, but you could see he was really doubting his role in his boys' lives now.

Kids grow out of things, sometimes before we're ready for it. Our role changes, and I think we go from 'needed' to 'being there'. As my kids grow up and evolve, my job is to be there in some shape or form.

Walking to school is a good metaphor for this change. What does walking them to school look like, now that you don't do it? What did they get out of that, and what did you get out of it? You're walking along with your child, you're enjoying the moment together, you're talking together about little things or maybe even big things. You're looking after your child. You're protecting them from the evils of the outside world. It's quality time.

So now that they're older, how do you get these things? How do you make them feel secure? How do you find moments when they can talk to you? Where are you getting your parent nourishment from, that closeness that you had so easily when they were little?

Kirsty: I agree with JK. His friend is still very much needed, but in a different way – and that's sometimes more of an adjustment for the parent than it is for the young person. It's interesting to think about what it is that you got out of that time when they were young. Because maybe the activities have changed, but the connection doesn't need to. It can just be found in different ways – sometimes more subtle, but still there.

There's a wealth of material about parenting during adolescence, and some of the recurring themes are *connectedness* and *consistency*. A sense of belonging – this is what the household, the home, provides as young people become more independent. They go out from home, but they come back to this safe base.

Whatever identity young people are trying out, out there in the big, wide world, they've always got this to come back to. It's their safe zone. As they try out these different identities and peer groups, some of them might go a bit haywire – but home is still solid. That consistency is so important – for the parent to be demonstrating that, whatever goes on out there, *I'm still here standing by you.*

They've got so much change to manage as they transition from primary to intermediate to high school, usually into bigger and bigger schools. In the best of worlds, their home base is stable and supportive.

Even if things aren't stable at home, or the relationship is challenging, it's a chance to work through the situation with them. That way you're modelling: *hard stuff happens, and here is how I'm managing or not managing. What can we do to get through this together?*

In psychology, we're always talking about teaching opportunities, or learning opportunities, and as kids negotiate through adolescence there are lots of opportunities to do this in a 'beside' way. By being open with your kids about the issues you confront in life, and modelling that openness, you are helping them be open about the issues in their lives.

When one of our own kids started college recently, he didn't necessarily need a hug from me any more, but I had to call him back and say, '*I* need the hugs now. But I promise I won't ask in front of your mates!' So, like with JK's friend, this heading off to school creates a bit of a separation issue for me. And it certainly raises the question: who are you in your child's life as they move into adolescence?

There's a part of this that is to do with accepting change. Accepting change is an important part of resilience. It's a normal part of life and it's inevitable, particularly through the adolescent years. We can make it easier on ourselves by exploring the true nature of the change, and seeking new things to put in its place.

By being open with our kids and exploring ways to maintain the connectedness, even through the changes of adolescence, the home base can be this safe base.

- Your role as a parent changes when your children enter adolescence – but you are still vitally important.
- Whatever identity young people are experimenting with out in the world, they benefit from coming back to a safe home base – a place of consistency and connectedness.
- By being open with your kids about the issues you confront in life, and modelling that openness, you help them be open about the issues in their lives.

53.
Resilience rests on relationships

Elliot: One of the most important things we can do to protect our children from depression is to raise them to be resilient. Resilience is about being able to recover readily from disappointments, frustrations or other misfortunes.

Historically, resilience was thought of as a personality type. But now it's seen as comprising personal attributes that you can develop. It's also seen as something that can be contained or encouraged in environments. Resilience rests, fundamentally, on relationships, as American psychologist Suniya Luthar has neatly put it.

Resilient social environments have high levels of trust (encouraging members of those communities to share their problems) and the capacity to act (which instils hope in those who seek help). Resilient children are much less likely to be overwhelmed by life's problems and challenges, and therefore are much less susceptible to depression.

A number of people have summarised what builds resilience. In *Help Me, I'm Sad*, David Fassler lists 'six essential principles' of raising a resilient child: loving and supporting the 'real' child; establishing predictability, availability and security; fostering open and honest communication; adopting a constructive and balanced approach to discipline; allowing children to experience life; and enhancing self-esteem. What is remarkable is how many of these principles rest on relationships. In that sense, we as parents can have a significant impact.

Much research has been done into the sorts of family structures and parental styles that are conducive to healthy development.

While there is plenty of public discussion of the dangers of divorce, low income or being in a one-parent family, in fact there are things that seem to be more important indicators of whether a young person will do well or not. Young people with parents who provide structures with clear but negotiable boundaries, consistent warmth, and consequences that are reasonable and not harsh generally do well. Families who deal with conflict constructively without violence, and set good role models for alcohol and other drug use also do better. Parents can act as a filter and have an influence on the type of friends their children have, their career choices and how much they value education. Young people take part in fewer risk-taking behaviours if they take part in collective family activities such as eating together, and collective out-of-school activities such as clubs, music, drama or sport.

Schools also have a vital part to play in developing resilient young people. Education that starts at an early age with an emphasis on teaching self-control, delayed gratification and developing relationships with adults to grow social skills have good evidence of effective outcomes. Schools that have high expectations, moderate classroom sizes, and in which teachers treat students with warmth, positive regard and support also have good outcomes academically. Better outcomes also occur, on average, when schools are smaller in size, have an emphasis on individual programmes not competition, and have mixed-ability rather than streamed classes – according to the Gluckman Report.

Resilience is not born out of 'hardening up' or being tougher. Resilience is born out of positive relationships that emphasise consistency, boundaries, reasonable expectations and consequences, communication and connectedness.

A story of resilience

Karl: I was 12 when I came to New Zealand, right before I started high school. I spoke English a little, but not the best. We came for my parents' work and to have a different life. They tried to prepare me, saying: 'It's not going to be easy. You are not going to have family or friends to start with. You have to socialise, and try and do things you wouldn't normally do.'

I was really excited – but it didn't strike me till I was here for a while that I wasn't going back. I started high school halfway through 2010. I was alone. I'd see the students in their friend groups, joking and laughing, having fun. I was alone and I felt different. I felt like an intruder.

I was very quiet. There were many times when I didn't know what to say, or I didn't understand the Kiwi slang, so I was really lost. It got bad to the point where I tried to isolate myself.

My parents would say 'Good day?' and I would say 'Yeah.' I wouldn't give them any details about my day. I didn't want them to feel bad.

I was sitting by myself and thinking about everything. I was angry with myself. I felt it was my fault I couldn't make friends.

I was also nice to myself, understanding myself: it wasn't easy, coming to a new country if English is your second language. I said to myself that it was going to take some time to fit in.

My eating habits went down. Noodles. The local bakery. Burger King. I guess I was using food as a comfort thing. I was about 40kg when we came – a small, skinny kid. And a year later I was about 57kg. I felt very unfit and big.

I had done athletics in Belgium – running, hurdles. I hadn't trained for a long time, but I saw they had an athletics club at school. I started going along, and after a while the coach started showing interest: he saw potential in me. It made me feel really good. When I ran I didn't think, *I'm in New Zealand*.

Now it's a very big part of my life. I still talk to my coach that I had in Belgium: the people I used to run with there are getting better, too, and I feel if I was to go back to Belgium and run with them, we could still run together.

I think athletics really helped, and people started to get to know me. It made socialising a lot easier. I met people at athletics I could talk to, and I made friends through that. Once I'd made one friend and talked to them, it made me more confident to talk to others. I built a strong group of friends after a while. Me and five others have been friends since the end of Year 9 and I always meet up with them at lunch and interval. We can talk about anything. I know people can go through a hard time and there's not a lot of things that can help, but talking is good.

Now I'm stronger than I was before. I've gone through that situation. I can say it was a hard time and I'm living happily.

If I was giving advice I'd definitely say, 'Talk to someone.' It could be a parent or a friend, a teacher or a dean. Then people understand your situation, and look out for you. Also, try and find something that can distinguish you: sport did that for me.

Listening to music helped me a lot. Sometimes the music of someone who's going through a hard time is helpful – it tells you, everyone has a hard time. You can say to yourself, *I'm having a hard time right now, but I'm not the only one.*

I knew I wasn't going to change without my own initiative to change. No one else was going to do it for me.

Know the change, accept it and get over the change: it is a process, a series of steps.

If another bad thing happened to me, I would feel bad and it would take me some time to acknowledge what was happening, but once I did acknowledge it I would be determined to overcome the situation.

I feel that after this situation, I can talk to my parents. When I was 12 I thought they might just tell me what I wanted to hear. They might try and talk it better. But life is hard and you have to work for certain things.

I will always be Belgian. But losing my accent helped me be Kiwi. I like New Zealand – the way people act and think positively around me. In Europe it is very hard to meet more people because there's so many people. Here, people are very friendly.

Kirsty: It would be great if there were two or three things that we could do to give our kids great self-esteem and the ability to 'bounce back' from tough times – that is, resilience. Unfortunately, there aren't just one or two techniques that hold the key to making our young person resilient or building their self-esteem.

On the other hand, there are lots of things we can do – we don't have to rely on just one or two – that can have a positive impact in these areas. Key to all of them is *us* – parents and caregivers – modelling healthy attitudes and behaviours. Our kids will learn more from what we do than what we say.

There are many building blocks for self-esteem and resilience that contribute to wellbeing. These include the following.

Social skills

- Good *communication skills* (surprise, surprise). Encourage your kids to share their feelings and what is going on in their world. Don't jump in to solve their problems – share ideas and assist with options, but show faith in them making good choices. You want them to know they can come to you. Listen, listen, listen.
- Teach your child good *social skills*: how to resolve issues that arise with friends, how to make friends, how to be a friend. Encourage them to think about how their behaviour might affect others.

Problem-solving and coping skills

- Introduce your child to a range of *coping strategies*. Model these yourself, and assist your child in discovering what works for them.
- Teach *structured problem-solving* and a flexible approach to things – define the problem, think of options, choose the best solution, try it out and then consider the outcome, and try something different if need be. Encourage a broad look at problems. Situations usually contain a bit of both good and bad. The online self-help programme for depression that JK fronts, called The Journal, has a fantastic module on this skill.
- Allow them to *experience failure* as well as success, and see the value in both. They need to develop resources for dealing with the difficult experiences in life – with you standing by them.
- *Model good coping* in your own life and identify other models – people who have overcome adversity or persisted in a course of action. Talk about these people who have overcome adversity. JK has become a touchstone in this sense for many adults who have struggled with mental illness.

Positive expectations, a sense of purpose and belief in the future

- *Celebrate successes* of all types – not just coming first, but doing something they found hard and getting a better result than the previous time.
- Assist your teen to *connect* with things that give them a sense of identity and purpose. Being part of a healthy community can be very helpful: good schools strive to provide this.
- Encourage a *'can do'* approach – we're good at that in New Zealand. Encourage kids to believe they can influence their outcomes.
- Love and support the child as they are, not as who you want them to be. Set up situations where they can gain confidence in the things they are good at, things that grow their strengths (not what *you* want their strengths to be). Encourage involvement in a variety of areas – the broader their experiences and areas they are involved in, the less the impact if one part of it goes awry.

Caring relationships

- Ensure some parental predictability and availability in the home, including times they know you will be around, and consistent household routines and rules.
- Have clear and consistent attitudes to boundaries and discipline that focus on the act, not the child.
- Create a sense of belonging in your immediate family, broader family, culture and community.
- Connect your young person with caring and supportive adults and mentors outside the family that they can turn to, if things aren't going well: aunties, uncles, grandparents, youth leaders, coaches, family friends.

Opportunities for participation

- Give your teen choices – include them in decision-making, encourage them to see options in situations and increase their sense of competence.

- Give them meaningful involvement and responsibility within the family, and in their community.

If you're like me, you look at this list and feel a sense of panic. Nobody can parent perfectly. But choose one element and focus on it for a week or month – see if it makes a difference for the young person, or in your household. Then move on to another. There are resources out there that assist with putting these things into place. The Parenting Place offers great parenting toolbox courses that cover a lot of these things: theparentingplace.com.

- Resilience is about being able to recover readily from disappointments, frustrations and other misfortunes.
- Resilience includes personal attributes that can be developed.
- Social environments or communities can also contribute to resilience: people can feel safe to share their problems with others, and confident that support will follow.
- Parents who provide structures with clear but negotiable boundaries, consistent warmth, and consequences that are reasonable and not harsh, have young people who generally do well.
- Focus on one of the building blocks of resilience at a time. See if it makes a difference, then move on to another.

54.
Wise people to help you through

Brook (youth worker): You can never lead anyone anywhere you haven't been yourself. How can a 17-year-old lead another 17-year-old out of crisis when they've never been in that crisis themselves? They can't. They can be a huge encouragement. Loving their friend unconditionally can be a glue that holds that young person and stops them from tipping over the edge. But they cannot lead them out of the hole if they haven't got out of holes themselves. We know this in life. If I have a crisis in my marriage, I don't go and talk to people who have the perfect marriage. I go and talk to the couple who I know had rocky times in their marriage and made it through. They had mastery of crisis; and I want to learn from people who have mastery of crisis.

Unfortunately, with young people who are struggling with mental health – which I consider, on a spectrum, is all young people, all human beings – their condition can be made worse if they don't have a wise and loving person to connect to. Obviously, there will be biological and chemical and medical reasons for the severity as well, but the presence of a loving parent, a loving friend, another human being who is there with grace and love and support, eases the pain – because they are sharing it with the person.

In this era that we're living in, many young people are not connected to close, supportive communities. History has led to the emergence of the nuclear man: the idea that *I am a solo system*.

Henri Nouwen wrote *The Wounded Healer* in 1978 – a premonition of the age to come. As we saw the nuclear family emerge in the 1960s and 70s, moving away from grandparents, aunties and uncles, he predicted that it would go from mum and dad and the kids, to *just me*. And he said that a key characteristic of the *just me*, or the nuclear man, would be that they would be inward-looking – when they looked for answers they would look in themselves – and this is really scary. Take a look on tumblr and watch what some young people are posting: their creative posts are all a reflection of what's happening inwardly to them. Rarely do you see in those posts the young people linking repetitively to an external wise voice. As Prime Minister John Key said, 'When young people have a problem, they Google it.'

The 'nuclear man' is an illusion, because even with the rise of individualism, and the idea that you can just look inwardly for the solutions to your own problems, there are a whole lot of colluding factors that come from your culture, your upbringing, your education, your family of origin, the random acts and experiences of your childhood that impact who you are today, and your response to actions and attitudes or opportunities or threats in life. We don't start on a level playing field.

55.
How do we talk to our kids?

Lou: Just knowing your parents are there for you if you want to talk. You might not want to sit down and have a huge discussion, and if they approach you to ask what's going on, you might want to do it in your own time. You might just want to have a casual conversation – casual, like not making a big deal, or creating a scene.

Ellen: Create opportunities for us to open up so that we don't feel we have to open up, but just have that option. But don't be offended if we don't right then.

Lou: Like, 'Do you want a chat?' If I say nah, then just open up the opportunity at another time, another day.

Jessica: Listening is a huge aspect of it. Just to have someone to listen and be there, even if they don't have the answers.

Scarlet: I want to be able to tell them stuff in confidence and them not jump down my throat. Being open and understanding is really good.

Olivia: When you do tell them stuff they should give a positive response even when it's not something they want to hear. The first time I told my mum something personal I felt awkward, and since then I haven't told her anything.

Jessica: Whenever my dad asks me if I'm OK and I say 'I'm fine', that's when I just want to shut him off. But then later I want to be asked again after I've had that time to myself to go over things.

JK: In the news the other night they were talking about an epidemic of people using sleeping pills and energy drinks together to get a high. This is our youth. It's not illegal. How do you protect your child from that? Ignore it? Talk about it?

For me this gets to the problem of what is good parenting. What are the rules? Some people think we should protect our kids from these things; but actually, the truth is, they're way ahead of us. I tend to think it's best to talk to them in a normal way about the things that they are actually seeing around them. But I might be getting it terribly wrong!

Anyway, I came home and said to the boys, 'I think this is a problem. What do you reckon?' Their mates are drinking alcohol and smoking marijuana at eighteen. I said, 'They'll probably try the sleeping pills and stuff then, won't they?' 'Yeah.' 'What do you reckon?' 'You should be able to have a good time without it.' 'Yeah, I reckon.' And we move on.

It's the same kind of thing with social media. My kids weren't allowed it for a long time. Now they use it, but we try and give it the balance that it should have. Sure, it's good for communication, but we try and make them realise that it's not human: you can't have 580 friends! How many of them would you cross the street to talk to? It's like everything else – it's education, a chance to talk about the issues, the pros and cons, highlighting some of the real negatives, and making them aware that it's an unreal world. You can't just leave it hanging out there and not talk about it.

From my point of view, all these things that go on in the real world are a chance to open the door to conversations.

Elliot: I agree: make it OK to talk about mental health and emotional issues in your household. Make it OK to talk about all the stuff that's really going on in the world – the hard stuff like drugs and suicide; and the things that make up the context of our kids' lives, like social media. I know it can be really hard, but remember in these conversations to listen to your kid's opinion with interest and without judging them, so that they'll feel comfortable about expressing themselves honestly. Try not to jump down their throat if they express an opinion that's different from yours or that alarms you. Use it as a chance to explore: 'Why do you think that?' Normalise those conversations so that, if ever something does go wrong, it won't be strange and unusual to be talking on that level.

Like JK's example with the energy drinks, you can use the media as a starting point – TV programmes, newspaper articles, things you hear on the radio or see on Facebook. You can say, 'It seems to me that this is really big, you know, lots of kids are self-harming. What do you think about that? Do you know any kids who do it? I'm really keen to talk to you if ever you feel that things are getting to this point . . .'

Sometimes it's helpful to have parents actually voicing in an upfront way that life can be hard for kids, or that schools are really stressful now, with all their demands for doing well academically and in competitive sport. Let them know that if it ever gets too much, they can talk to you – and if not to you, then that's fine, but to someone else, and you can help them to find some support. That kind of acknowledgment can be very meaningful.

It's good if these conversations aren't too big and heavy. I like JK's example of the energy drink conversation – very short, but it was enough: the boys knew he was interested in their opinion, that he was thinking of them, and it opened the door for them to talk more if they wanted.

We have already mentioned commonground.org.nz as a good place to go for ideas about having conversations. It's a great New Zealand website that outlines ways to get talking about a wide variety of challenges our young people face.

- Make it OK to talk about mental health and emotional issues in your household.
- Things that go on in the real world provide an opportunity to open the door to conversations with your kids. Use media coverage of issues as a starting point.
- Listen to your kids' opinions with interest, and without judging them.
- Commonground.org.nz is a good website that has lots of ideas about starting conversations with teens.

56.
Open the door

Scarlet: When I'm going through a tough time, I appreciate it that my mum does practical things to help me, like, I come home and she's made my bed; or there's a nice cooked meal; or if I've got a tournament going on and she gets stuff ready for me, it takes those other pressures out of the way. Sometimes she'll ask me if I want to talk, saying 'What's up?' But if I don't want to talk she'll let me ride it out a bit. It's like, 'OK, when you're ready we can talk about things.'

Jim: It starts at a young age. If they're talking to you about stuff like this at a young age, then as you get older you feel more comfortable.

Flora: My parents started talking to me when I was older, and that was fine for me. I didn't want to say anything when I was younger. I just didn't need to.

Jim: Don't bombard us with shit. Don't not talk to us for three months then bombard us with questions.

Kylie: You have to drop the lecturing role. Don't give me the PowerPoint presentation.

Kate: A 'do' would be: give random bursts of attention. It lets me know they're interested and it's like, they do care.

JK: With my son I go, 'Hey boy, what's up?' And he says, 'Good.' I don't blame him for that; I blame me. How can I get a dialogue going with him? What am I doing wrong?

Kirsty: JK isn't doing anything wrong. He's doing the right thing – he's noticing that maybe something's troubling his son, and he's asking him about it. He's not getting the answer he's hoping for – not at this stage, anyway – but it's important not to have expectations of these conversations. You *might* get a conversation, but it's quite likely you'll get a shrug-off in the first instance. 'Don't be dumb . . . I'm fine . . . leave me alone.' But what you've done is you've opened the door for that conversation. You've let them know that you're willing to have it if they ever need to have it. It's about creating an environment where it's OK to talk.

Don't be afraid to talk to your kids when you have that feeling that things aren't quite right. Tell them what you've noticed: 'I'm getting a feeling that maybe something is worrying you at the moment . . .'; 'I've noticed you've been a bit withdrawn – are you feeling OK?' Once you've opened the door, it gives you a base to go back to: 'I commented the other day that you didn't seem yourself; I'm still noticing that and I'm getting quite worried about you . . .'

Trust yourself. Have those conversations and keep having them. Don't doubt yourself or give up, just because you get the grunt.

You might need to accept that your child doesn't want to talk to you at this stage, and that's when it can be good to enlist the support of someone else – a special aunt or uncle or older cousin or a family friend they may be more open to. Tap them on the shoulder and say: 'I may be totally overreacting, but it would be great if you could just check in to see how they're going because they may be more open to talking with you.'

Elliot: I agree – it's so important to normalise the process. Trust your instincts, ask your questions, but factor in that you may well get knocked back. And the two key things for parents to take on board are: don't take it personally; and don't assume that you're doing something wrong in asking, and go hands-off.

You're never going to make it worse by asking. Even if you ask in the 'perfect' way you still might not get an answer. It's just the way it can be sometimes.

Kirsty: A colleague of mine made a lovely statement about this: 'You don't know what you're preventing by asking the question.' It's a statement that comes from the suicide prevention sector, but it also applies really well if you've got concerns about depression.

You'll never know what might have happened if you hadn't asked. But given that a classic part of depressive thinking is: *People don't care about me . . . no one would care if anything happened to me . . . I'm worthless . . . I'm useless . . .*, the very fact that you are asking concerned questions contradicts some of those thoughts that they might be having. That's immensely powerful, and even if the response is to shrug it off, you've given them some evidence against the depressive thinking by conveying that you do care.

It was interesting how, when JK asked the group of high school students what he should do if he was concerned about a young person, how to have a conversation with them and what they would most want to hear – they all had different ideas. Some wanted him to talk with their friends, some didn't; some wanted to talk at home; some wanted to talk when out. But there was one thing in common: all of them wanted you to start the conversation. All of them said they would want their parent to ask; and all of them wanted their parent to listen and not judge or lecture. All of them acknowledged that they might not be in the mood when you first ask and so you'd just get a grunt in reply, but all of them wanted you to ask again. None of them said they wanted their parent to come up with the right answer.

So – ask, listen, don't judge, ask again. It sounds pretty easy, but it actually takes a lot of effort! Practise – you may get a few laughs and startled looks from your young person, but give it a try!

- If you suspect something is troubling your young person, ask them about it. But don't have expectations for the conversation.
- Don't worry if you don't get much of an answer – you've opened the door for the conversation, and they know you're there if they want to talk.
- It's about creating an environment where it's OK to talk: one that is heavy on listening, and light on lecturing and judging!
- Ask them again later.
- It's not about having the right answer. It's about caring enough to ask and to listen if they do want to talk.

57.
'I'm like a private investigator'

Claudia (Nakita's mum): The big thing I'd say is to really have your finger on the pulse of your kid. A lot of kids are going down the slippery slope and their parents don't have any idea. So, instead of being at the top of the cliff, parents end up being the ambulance at the bottom, with a child that's got so far into depression and the parents never saw it happening. These kids are our responsibility and we need to be really looking for signs.

If I have a gut instinct that something is wrong with my kids, I'm like a private investigator. I don't stop. I don't take their word for it. As a parent, you know your kid. You gave birth to them, you've lived with them all these years. You should know if they're happy or sad. It's your instinct, so don't believe it when they say nothing's wrong.

Get into all the corners of their lives and try to find out. Not in an overbearing way, but try to work it out. *She's coming home depressed – well, who's she hanging out with?* Piece things together. Don't brush it off. Really seek the answers.

'Nothing's wrong', 'It's just one of those days' – these are brush-offs. Inside, the kid is often thinking, *I wish you'd ask me again; I will tell you but I can't now.* So take time to be with them, and do ask again, in different ways, using different words. Often a key word that you use will suddenly break them open.

Talk to their friends and their siblings, their teacher. Get a picture of what's going on. The kid will say, 'Don't say anything to the teacher.' But I think, *you're my responsibility and if I don't say anything then nothing will change*. I go and talk to the teacher. I say to my kids: 'We need to be that for you guys. We're doing it because we love you. I'll stand up for you when no one else will.'

Often they end up saying, 'Thanks for talking to the teacher. It has made a difference.'

58.
Emotional intelligence – but then what?

JK: Call it gut instinct, emotional intelligence, intuition, whatever – it's that thing we have a lot of when it comes to our kids. Whether we trust it or not is another matter. In fact, it's all too easy to overlook it. Gut instinct, by its very nature, is a feeling that comes from our subconscious, and for various reasons – a culture that is very keen on science and empirical evidence rather than anything that is unseen; a culture that is not very emotionally expressive; or the fact that we are all very busy making ends meet and living our busy lives – we either don't even register those inner feelings that are trying to tell us something is wrong, or we tell ourselves we're imagining it.

Layla (Christie's mum): I took her to the doctor because I was worried she was losing weight. I asked the doctor then, 'Do you think she's underweight?' She said not to worry, 'Her BMI's a bit on the low side but I don't like to be too judgmental of kids at this age because they all grow and develop at different rates.' I guess as a parent you want to hear there's not a problem, so I went away feeling a bit uneasy, but allowed myself to be reassured.

JK: Well, maybe because I've been to hell and back, I've learned to trust my gut instinct. When I walk into a room of people, or when I'm with my kids, I look and I observe and I get a feeling about how they are emotionally, and I react to that. I call that my EQ – my emotional intelligence.

After the Asian tsunami of 2004 there was lots of evidence that elephants and other animals had sensed it was coming and escaped to higher ground. In one case in Thailand, a tour party of eight elephants bolted for high ground, charging through the jungle with frightened tourists clinging on for dear life. Soon after that, the waves struck below, killing thousands along the coast. The elephants knew. Somehow they picked up the signals and they acted. They followed their instinct. They didn't wait around.

I try to listen to my gut and not my brain, and I trust myself to follow that instinct. Sometimes it scares me, but I'll follow it regardless.

My older son, Niko, is 18 now. He's externally boisterous; he's usually the least of my worries because he's always been so confident. But internally I was getting a feeling . . . maybe I needed to dig a wee bit deeper and just make sure his confidence was real? But how do I do that? I asked questions: 'What are you worried about?' I can sense there's something, but he won't answer. 'Good,' he says. 'Nothing.'

But I'm glad I got the feeling and I'm glad I asked, because a few nights later we were all out, and at the end of the evening he came and found me and he said, 'Drive home with me, Dad.' I never usually do, because I come home with Fiorella, but he'd come looking for me. That was the message that he wanted to chat about some stuff, and driving home together he could tell me what was going on.

But this brings me to my problem. So, my EQ got me asking him what was wrong – but what next? This is my fear as a parent: that I don't have the knowledge to really help him with the right answers. How do I give him the answers that will help him find the confidence he needs?

Kirsty: It's really tricky, because as a parent we want to be there for our kids and have the answers for them – to say the right things that will help them through life. This is what we tend to do when they're young and the 'right answers' are easier to come by. But as they get older and more independent and the situations get more complex, our role needs to shift.

We can't give them the 'right answer' any more, partly because it's not all that easy to come by – there's seldom one 'right' answer or 'right' thing to say. But most importantly, if we keep stepping in with the 'right answer', what will they do when we're not there to give it to them? Our role needs to move in to being there for them, having tricky conversations with them, being a sounding board and helping them to problem-solve. It's a very important thing: it's not always our role to answer the question and to make it right. Sometimes we have to say, 'It's not easy and there's no simple answer or you'd have figured it out for yourself.'

Problem-solving might involve moving through questions such as: 'What do you think the options might be? How would that work out? What other options might there be? Which one do you want to try? What would help or hinder that? What are the good and not so good things about each option? Is there anything I can do? Let's touch base in a day/week and see if that's made a difference. Let me know if it gets any worse in the meantime. Good on you, this is hard – I'm proud of you.'

We are shifting into teaching our young person how to solve issues that come their way, either internal or external. We aren't abandoning them in this; we're walking alongside them, acknowledging their experience, being a sounding board, suggesting options, teaching them skills, and increasing their self-confidence in managing what life throws at them.

The UK *Good Childhood Report 2013*, which surveyed over 42,000 young people, highlighted the importance of choice in adolescence wellbeing. The degree of choice that young people perceived they had impacted on their sense of wellbeing. Depression and anxiety, along with the associated agency involvement, identity uncertainty and worries about the future can all feel like they are robbing a young person of choice. In your conversations with your young person, through the problem-solving that you encourage them to do, find ways to help them see choice in what they do and in what lies ahead. Having choice gives hope.

- As our kids get older, we won't always have the right answers.
- Our role becomes to be a sounding board and to support our kids to problem-solve their way forward.
- Having choice enhances wellbeing.

59.
Around the dinner table – connectedness

JK: We eat together as a family almost every night – at least five nights a week. We set the table, the television goes off, we sit down. We wait for each other, too. We eat when the last person's got home and that might be nine o'clock – Italians eat a lot later than New Zealanders. For me that's really fundamental.

You are the parent, you create the environment.

I do feel that New Zealand has lost its way in some respects. We have this perception of ourselves that we're a family-oriented country, but we've actually become a career-driven, Americanised country where there's a big emphasis on what car you drive and what you happen to be earning. The values have become more individual, and the emphasis has shifted away from kids and families.

I know it's hard for families – often two people have to work, or they have to work very long hours or shifts. But to me, someone has to be there when the kids come home from school. It's a fundamental. I don't care if it's the mother or the father – someone has to be there. We've got to make time for kids, and we've got to make time for families.

In Italy, where I've lived for many years and where my kids have spent most of their lives, they do lunch. You go to school or work from 8 a.m. till 1.30, then you have lunch and siesta till 3.30, and then you go back to work till 7 p.m. So that tradition creates the family time. For those two hours in the middle of every day you're with your family. Lunch is for your family; at night you can do what you want. Obviously we don't do that here because school and work schedules don't allow it, but we make sure we eat together every night. A solid family home makes society better.

It's not just at home that we eat together. Until I came to New Zealand I had never been out for dinner without my kids. We go everywhere together, and the kids become more rounded. If you take them out when they're five, they can sit round the table at 14 and know when to speak and when not to speak, and they can be part of the conversation. They learn how to socialise with adults. But here we're asked out and it's 'no kids'. My wife asks me three times 'Why aren't the kids coming?' I have to answer, 'I don't know.'

Elliot: There is research evidence – large studies from overseas and in New Zealand – that eating meals together as a family is associated with positive outcomes for young people. It seems such a tiny thing, doesn't it? Even after controlling for other forms of family connectedness, ethnicity, deprivation and the ways parents communicate, frequent family meals have been associated with less substance use, fewer depressive symptoms, less suicidal ideation, fewer risk-taking behaviours and better grades.

The Youth'12 Report found that 62 percent of students reported that their family had eaten meals together five or more times in the past week. So about 40 percent didn't.

Family meals are a basic of family connectedness, and connectedness is a major cornerstone of resilience and mental wellness. Resilience rests, fundamentally, on relationships, remember! It makes sense, doesn't it? Not only is sharing food one of the most fundamental of all human activities, but sitting at a table together is sometimes the only time in the day when people have the time and opportunity to check in with each other. Sometimes mealtime conversation is not much more than a round-up of the day ('What did *you* do today?'), but sometimes a conversation is sparked that stimulates everyone and leaves all family members feeling engaged and positive about each other. Connected.

'Social connectedness is protective for young people,' says Professor Gluckman in the Gluckman Report. He was talking about suicide prevention, but the point is true across the board.

Connectedness is vital in the struggle against depression in particular, as the sense of belonging is in contradiction to the isolation and negative self-talk of that illness (*no one loves me; I'm unlovable*).

If we can create occasions for connecting with our young people we will not only build stronger families and communities, we will greatly increase our chances of noticing when something is going wrong for them.

The Mental Health Foundation (mentalhealth.org.nz) and The Parenting Place (theparentingplace.com) have lots of suggestions for ways in which we can connect with each other and our communities, including the following.

Within the family

- Do things together, and make opportunities to talk or just to 'be' together (driving to sports, dropping them off at a friend's, going to the supermarket/shops, fishing, walking the dog, cooking dinner or baking, playing cards or a board game).
- Have positive family rituals and traditions (birthday celebrations or special times of the year, ways to celebrate when someone has done well, places you go together, eat together, have fun together).
- Do a 'round' during family meals of 'best thing that happened today', 'funniest thing that happened today', 'hardest thing that happened today', 'most interesting thing that happened today', 'something I'm grateful for today' (take turns choosing the topic).
- Record special family events through photos, scrapbooks or a memories box that your young person can add to and browse through to reinforce their belonging.
- Have family movie nights, family games nights, family anything nights (be creative!).
- Have meals with other families – a bring-a-pizza-topping night, or shared fish and chips.
- If your immediate family is in turmoil, make an effort to connect your young people with supportive extended family

through get-togethers, coffee, movies, activities or online (for instance, Skype).

Within your community

- Connect your young person with community groups and associated supportive adults (e.g. sports clubs, scouts and guides, youth groups, arts groups or church groups).
- Promote a sense of belonging within your cultural group. Encourage your young person to explore their cultural background and ways they can connect with this. Do this alongside them through cultural groups, opportunities to use their language, etc.
- Take part as a family in community events (neighbourhood clean-ups, school events, cultural events, art and other events) – check out your local newspaper for what's on.

We appreciate that young people, particularly in their teenage years, may well be less than enthusiastic at times about engaging in some of the things you suggest! Start young, make it a part of being in the family, and persist – particularly if your teen is unwell, as the symptoms of depression and anxiety can make it very hard for them to engage. A number of the young people we interviewed noted that they were reluctant at the time to engage in things with their family or others, but that these things did make a difference in the end.

Be realistic and find out what works for your family. Get ideas from your young people (when they are in a forthcoming mood) about things they would like to do together, and start there. Building connectedness and belonging takes time and effort, particularly if it feels like you are starting from scratch. But the outcomes make it well worth the effort.

- Research shows that kids from families who regularly eat meals together have less substance use, fewer depressive symptoms, less suicidal ideation, fewer risk-taking behaviours and better grades.
- Family meals are a basic of family connectedness, and connectedness is a major cornerstone of resilience and mental wellness.
- Find ways to connect within your family and your community, to build that sense of belonging for your kids.

60.
Going out for pizza

JK: Let's say I have noticed some mood changes. You might be bitchy with me, you might be in your room, headphones on, listening to Eminem . . . How do I, if I'm the perfect dad, initiate a conversation?

Sophie: Don't get mad about it. Don't get mad that I'm snapping at you. Just keep calm.
Jim: Don't be like, 'Why are you so antisocial? Why are you sitting in your room?' Because it's like piling on the negative.

JK: What would you like to hear?

Sophie: You could ask them to do something that you know they like, like go out for dinner.
Flora: Like take them out for pizza.

JK: So I say, 'Wanna go out for pizza tonight?'

Flora: Yep.

JK: What if I get a no?

Jim: Sometimes you're just not in the mood. Everyone goes out and you're just bottling it up.
Sophie: Don't take siblings with you, because then they're getting the attention as well. Sometimes, you just want attention. Also, you don't want the rest of the family sitting there listening.

Olivia: If it was me, I wouldn't want to go somewhere and eat and talk about my problems, because if it was actually serious I wouldn't want to open up in that public area. I would rather as a family go out for food and then get back in a better mood. Then your parents could come into your room and talk about it.

61.
Quality time – whose definition of 'quality'?

Jessica: I've got quite a big family, and in tough times I can feel really lonely. There's so much happening at home, you can get lost in it. There are so many people there, they might not see the signs of what's happening, cos there are so many people to look after, and then you can just . . . drift away.

JK: It's an interesting thing, the idea of 'quality time'. I get that parents need to make sure they have time to strengthen themselves and also their relationship. But for Fiorella and me, our strength is our kids and we want them around us all the time. We find time for us, but our perfect day is having the kids around all the time and we're doing stuff. We'd rather have everyone in the house. If they want friends, we'd rather have them around at ours. We make space. And then we don't get involved, we're just there. Well, Fiorella gets really involved, asking questions, but I just take a back seat. That's how we like to do things.

Every stage in life is different. I'm surfing with my kids now. We've got the beach house at Waihi, so we do that a lot. The last day of summer I was out the back with my two sons, we were surfing and they were yahooing, having a great time, just enjoying surfing as I know it, and I was out there with them enjoying it, too. Each age has its stage. I guess for me it's about creating a want: that they *want* to do that with me.

For me it's about getting the balance right at home so they feel they can discuss or talk about anything, right or wrong. And that they want to be home. So this is still their sanctuary.

Kirsty: There's a fascinating statistic from the Youth'12 Report that shows less than half of high-school-age kids felt they spent enough time with their parents. It's actually quite poignant – but I find it fascinating because it's so counterintuitive. And because it describes a really simple way for parents to step into their kids' lives.

That statistic is contrary to the idea that in adolescence kids want to separate themselves completely from their parents. While forming their own identity is a key task of this phase of life, I think that can sometimes be misinterpreted by parents as *we should back off*; or *we have to let them be independent*; or *they'd much rather be hanging out with their friends then spending time with us*. Yet here we have all these kids saying they don't get enough time with their parents.

There were some really great, optimistic stats in the Youth'12 Report: 81 percent said their family members got along well or very well, and 69 percent of students had fun with their families often or a lot. The overwhelming majority – 93 percent – felt their mother and/or father cared a lot about them. But only about half the students said they got enough time with their mothers most of the time; and 37 percent said they got enough time with their fathers. The reasons for not spending enough time with their parents were that they were at work, or busy with housework and other children or family members. With fathers, there was the added significant reason that he didn't live with them.

That's as strong a call as any that kids are hungry for their parents. It certainly doesn't have to be anything big and meaningful – it might just be that you get everyone together to watch a TV programme after dinner or go for a walk around the neighbourhood. Just being together, sharing an experience, is the key thing.

This brings us to the idea of 'quality time' that JK mentions. Can a small amount of intensely shared time with your kids make up for less quantity of time spent together? This is a hotly debated area; and probably a mixture of both is the best option. Perhaps a more important way to look at it is: whose version of 'quality' is it?

As adults, our version of quality time with someone might be having a good heart to heart and really getting an idea of what's going on in their heads; but a kid's version of quality time is probably more along the lines of just hanging. *Oh, I just watched TV with Dad; Mum and I went and had a milkshake while we were getting those socks I needed for school* – just being with someone, knowing you were there in the background while they were doing their homework and they could chat to you if they wanted, but they didn't have to.

It's to do with *presence*. When you are doing something with them, are you engaged in that activity with them? Are you in the same headspace? Are you available to talk within that task if they wanted to – or is your headspace somewhere else?

It's quality time if I'm engaged with the young person in whatever this activity is, whether it's fixing something together, or driving somewhere, or sitting in a café. I'm not checking my texts; I'm not driving and talking to someone on the phone at the same time; I'm not driving and they're listening to their music through headphones. It's not just about being in the same physical space; it's about being in the same headspace. I might say: 'Let's put your music on over the car stereo so I can listen, too' – and I don't say it's terrible!

Elliot: You're not going to get far if you sit your child down, fix them with a serious look and say, 'So, how's it *really* going?' It's way too confronting. It's a lot better to be doing things alongside, and just open up the opportunities for a conversation. I think especially with boys, having a chat as you're driving along is easier for them. They don't have to look at you, and you can't look at them.

- Less than half of high-school-age kids feel they spend enough time with their parents.
- Quality time with kids is in part about *presence* – about just being around and being together in the same headspace.

62.
Somebody to lean on

JK: Learning to trust in friendship, to not be afraid of what people would think when they found out what was really going on for me, was part of my journey to wellness. If I'd been able to talk to my friends sooner, I'm sure I would have found help much earlier.

Hannah: My friends were exceptionally important – they kept me engaged in the real world. They were just my friends. They didn't talk in technical language or diagnoses, they were not my therapists, they just continued being my friends and they were just the best thing. One friend is sick with anxiety and depression at the moment, and so it's my chance to just be her friend and try and make her go to the doctor.

There's not an easy answer. When someone is sick you kind of think, *oh, we'll just hang out and go to the movies.* But actually it's hard and you can feel that everything's changed and your relationship is not the same. But you almost have to pretend it is still the same.

Having a chat, a conversation, making a time for it and planning it. Talking about something unrelated to medication. Something that you're familiar with that you can chat about. Mum used to read the newspaper to come up with conversation when I was eating. Or if having a conversation was too much, then watching a movie or a TV series, one that you've seen before, maybe, so it's even less effort. Some people might say, 'Go out for coffee', but that was too hard. Other people had to make the plans and show up and do most of the talking.

Something that made a huge impact on my recovery was my friends talking to me about their plans after they left school – the universities they applied to, their gap year. I wasn't doing that – I needed to start thinking about my life, and I wasn't in a position to do that. It was hugely motivating hearing about what they were up to.

The other thing that was helpful was invitations. Even if people knew I was going to say no they kept inviting me to coffee or movies or dinner. I've heard that it's really hard to keep reaching out when you're not getting any response, but it was really helpful. I'd get a text and I'd think, *they still care. I'm still part of the group. There's something waiting for me.*

My friend wrote me a quote: 'Every day will not be good but there will be some good in every day', and I've still got it, and that is so true with mental illness. So often every day is awful, but there's one little comment or conversation.

Moana: I think having good friendships with your son or daughter's friends, being able to talk to their friends without your son or daughter being there. I generally have good relationships with my friends' parents.

Scarlet: Inclusiveness, especially for teenagers and young people. Even if you don't admit it, being included and part of something is really important, because it gives you that sense of belonging. Also, having people who keep you moving and keep you going is important – a friend who says, 'Let's go and do some training together.' Keeping them going in some way is important. Getting through a tough time is not always about addressing the issue right away; it might just be about being there, and reminding them of the other things they've got in their life.

Jessica: Communication is important, but it doesn't always have to be between the parent and the child. It could be between the child and another adult, like a youth worker or a friend's parent.

Kirsty: It's useful to think about the variety of ways that someone can be there for you – and to get your young person to think about that, too – when you're looking at who can be there to support them. There are different ways in which they (and we) can 'connect' with people, and gain different things from these connections. Supports can include:

- someone they can talk with about what is going on for them
- someone who distracts them from the difficult things they are struggling with

- someone who makes them laugh
- someone who has a similar interest
- someone who connects them to their past – their belonging
- someone who connects them to their future – their possibilities
- someone who encourages them and makes them feel good about themselves
- someone who supports a way to be well (for instance, exercises with them).

Mel (Hannah's mum): Against Hannah's wishes and unbeknown to her, I chose eight of her good friends and rang their parents and told them she'd been diagnosed with anorexia, and that I believed they had a role to play in her recovery. 'I'm approaching you to see if you're prepared to be involved.' The next morning I had eight mothers and daughters around this table. They all turned up, weeping. They were fantastic, and absolutely integral for Hannah's recovery. I told her I'd done it and she said, 'Thank you so much.' She couldn't have done it herself.

I knew it was best for everybody to get it out in the open. I recommend, though, that you choose the friends carefully, and bring in the parents if you trust them. There is such a stigma around mental illness, and that stigma is such a barrier to recovery. That's why, as soon as I felt confident enough, I went quite public and I said, 'We want people to talk *to* us, not *about* us.'

It's really important to find support among other people going through what you're going through, to share experiences and resources, and to remind you that you're not alone. If no one talks about it, everyone thinks they're the only one dealing with it.

As soon as Hannah started coming right I reached out to meet other people. Now there are quite a few of us, and I find it really helpful. We say to each other, 'It's absolutely awful, isn't it, but in the scheme of things what you're going through is normal, so put aside all thoughts of giving up.'

Kirsty: Your teen may have difficulty reaching out to their friends when they are unwell, and their friends may worry about the appropriateness of connecting with your teen. It might be appropriate for you to make the connections for them.

- Good friendships are protective. Foster your teen's healthy relationships, and get to know their friends.
- When your child is ill, they need your support and the support of their friends.
- Support comes in different forms.

63.
Build a community

JK: It might be the brother, the sister, the aunty, the friend – it doesn't matter. We need people around us to support us, to stand by us.

We're lucky to have a big extended family. We were together the other day and all the nieces and nephews were there. We were all there as brothers and sisters, and all our next generation were there, talking and laughing. We're very much in each other's lives. Life changes around us, but we're really close. We know each other intimately, so we can relax, no inhibitions, and we laugh and take the mickey. This is the kids' go-to group, their family, their cousins.

I love Claudia's suggestion that if you haven't got a close extended family around you, actively go out and build yourself a community. Do it deliberately.

Claudia (Nakita's mum): We have a lot of people around us. Nakita has grandparents, godparents, youth workers who are all giving her the same messages we are. Our community has helped us . . . But unfortunately a lot of people don't have this and are isolated. I advise parents to go out and consciously build a community around their kids. Be discerning about who you choose. These people will support you and support your kids.

Catherine (Sean's mum): I'm not a 'Christian' Christian, but I feel I practise Christian principles and have some sort of spirituality. Tied up with that is my belief that our lives unfold the way they're supposed to. And if that life throws us some shoddy stuff, it's how we deal with it that's important. Along those lines I've recently read a really good quote: *Life* *isn't about waiting for the storm to pass. It's about learning how to dance in the rain.*

I have a Christian friend who put Sean on the prayer chain at her church. She told me there was one lady in particular who always asked after him. So, who knows? Maybe these people who've been 'intercessioning' *may* have helped Sean. Maybe they put his new girlfriend in his way? Maybe they've decided that enough's enough, now. Maybe the powers that be, whoever they are, have decided to give Sean a break – or they've decided his parents deserve some sleep!

- If you haven't got a close extended family around you, actively go out and build yourself a community. Look to find one that feels right for you and your young person.

PART EIGHT
Wellness is Everyday

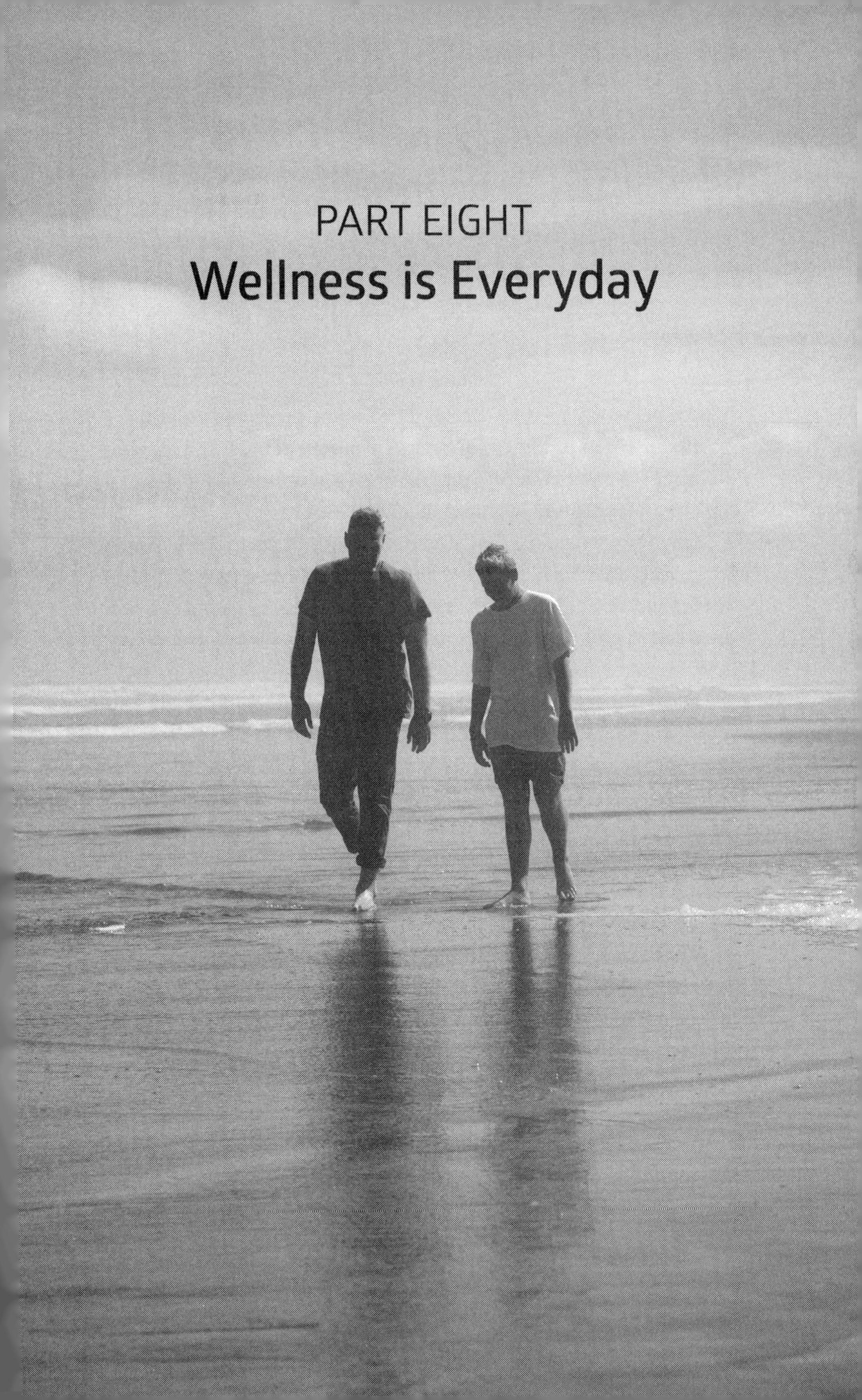

64.
Pathways to wellness

JK: I've been well now for nearly 20 years, but I never take it for granted. When it comes to mental health, wellness isn't an end-point, it's a process. A lifelong process. You're not going to wake up one morning and be cured. It's a journey.

One thing coaching teaches you is the importance of having a plan. You can have all the talent, but you need everything in place – tactics and strategies – so that no matter what happens you can stay on track. A good plan gives you freedom, so that when everything hits the fan you go back to plan.

For me it works like that with depression. If you have a plan you can cope with whatever life throws at you.

Your wellness plan begins with building self-knowledge and self-awareness. What are the things that stress you? How does your body feel when it's getting stressed? What helps you to chill when things get stressful? What do you enjoy doing? For me it might be taking a few minutes to sit outside, or going for a swim. *You* need to find the things that make *you* feel good.

There are no rules about this. Your things will be different from my things. For me, having a coffee – sipping it slowly, really tasting it – is one of the things I love. It's a little thing that anchors me in the moment, and I create a moment to consciously enjoy. But you might hate coffee . . . And that's the fun part of this: getting out there and finding the things you love to do.

That's what I did: I went on a fun journey to find out what keeps me mentally relaxed. I just kept trying stuff. I tried everything with an open mind. I found I'm an active relaxer. I'm not good at sitting still doing nothing. But reading, playing the guitar, going to the shops and selecting good food and bringing it home and cooking it for my family – those things I love and they bring me peace.

Wellness is everyday. What does that mean? It means finding the simple, everyday pleasures that tell you who you are in a positive way, and building those things into your life so that every day you are feeding those aspects of yourself that you enjoy. It's a work in progress; a constant work in progress. When I'm under pressure I come back to my wellness plan. I check in with myself about the thing I'm stressed about. I analyse why I'm stressed.

It's like when I was depressed and Michael Jones gave me the lifeline of telling me I had a good heart. I could come back to that idea: *I feel awful . . . but I've got a good heart.* Now, if I'm stressed, I come back to baseline questions: What can I control? Am I doing the best I can? What's the right thing to do? If it's a professional matter I'm worried about, I keep it in its professional box. I don't let it into the boxes I have for my personal happiness, or my family life.

And in my life, I come back to baseline wellness strategies: if I'm feeling a bit under pressure, I know I need to slow down, do one of my relaxation things – go for a swim, play my guitar, have a nice breakfast and really focus on tasting the food. Get together with people I love and do some laughing.

These are the pathways to wellness. They stop me treading the road back to depression and anxiety.

Helene: I'm much more aware now of when I'm going off track. The time when everything went wrong, it was a surprise to me that it had got to that point, but looking back I can see it was obvious. Now I can recognise the signs instantly. That nervous butterfly tummy; or headaches – it's the physical sign that things are getting on top of me, that I've taken things too far and I need to stop and take a step back.

Kirsty: It's not really surprising that people don't understand and are so nervous of mental illness. It's not just because of the extremely rare incidences of bad outcomes (death or harm to others) that get sensationalised in the media. It's that for so long – right up until the past couple of decades – it was considered a life sentence where all hope for a satisfying, ordinary life was gone, and where people were consigned to the margins of society, often shut away in institutions as 'mental patients'.

Thank goodness, there has been a massive change in the way mental illness is seen and treated. In the United States, the former First Lady Rosalynn Carter, who led the 1979 President's Commission on Mental Health, said in 2003 that the biggest change she'd seen over the previous 25 years was that the concept of 'recovery' was transforming the field of mental health. 'Today, the reality is that the overwhelming majority of people with mental illnesses will recover if only they get help,' she told a recent symposium.

Today, there is a world of hope, where before there was little.

Elliot: In the mental health field we refer to 'recovery-oriented treatment', which says it is possible to have a life with illness. Mental health professionals recognise that in some cases there may be no cure: some people with depression, anxiety or other mental illnesses may have to manage some symptoms indefinitely. This doesn't mean they can't lead full lives with positive identities, meaningful relationships and a sense of purpose. Within mental health the term 'recovery' is increasingly used to mean living well in the presence or absence of illness. It is recognised that people with chronic physical illnesses such as asthma can make adaptations and manage, without the condition defining them. Mental illness is no different.

So, in mental health we talk about recovery rather than cure. Wellness is everyday, as JK says. It's not an endpoint; rather, it's a constant state of being.

Recovery is about knowing yourself: recognising that you have the potential to become depressed or anxious, and building up the strengths in yourself so you can meet life's challenges in a healthy way. Good therapy will spend a lot of time on this.

Your young person should cover the following with their therapist and/or others close to them (including you).

- ways to recognise when things aren't going well for them – their personal 'warning signs'
- times when they might be more vulnerable (exams, relationship issues)
- what their strategies are for managing this, including supports they can go to and things they can do on their own
- what keeps them well, and what makes them strong or gives them peace when they are stressed

A lot of people find the knowledge of themselves that they gain through the recovery process makes them stronger and happier than they were before they became ill. We call this 'positive psychology' or post-traumatic growth – the idea that on the other side of trauma can lie something worthwhile; that something really bad happens but, because you find a way to deal with it, you grow as a person. It's really a fancy new title for an ancient idea. Religion and literature have for centuries, if not millennia, pointed out the role of human suffering in bringing people closer to wisdom, truth and God.

I certainly don't want to romanticise the terrifying experience of going through, or watching your child go through, depression or anxiety; and I'm sure most parents would say they would rather it had never happened. We all want to rescue our children from hurt, don't we? But interestingly, every young person we interviewed for this book said that, while they hated being depressed, they felt it had been an important part of shaping who they are, and making them a stronger, more empathetic person.

In the medical sense, we can't talk about a 'cure' for depression and anxiety, or for other mental illness, but we can talk about recovery; and we can talk about living really well – even exceptionally well – in the presence of mental illness.

- Most people with mental illness will recover if they get help.
- Recovery is about knowing yourself – recognising that you have the potential to become depressed or anxious; building up your strengths to meet life's challenges in a healthy way; and learning to live with your illness if you have to.
- Wellness isn't an endpoint, it's a process.

65.
Things that make you feel good

Scarlet: It's not like a one size fits all. You can't just take one person's experience and say that it's going to work for your own kind of lifestyle.
Helene: I plan nice things for myself so I've got those to look forward to – things like going to a movie or getting a pedicure or having a weekend away. I try really hard now to make sure that I have down time, or time that's just for me. I used to find it difficult to say no because I wanted to please everyone. I'm a lot more comfortable with saying no and not feeling I have to explain, justify or make up for it. By saying no and taking time for myself I avoid getting stressed and anxious.

JK: Every day I go to work, I'm a father, I'm a husband, I'm a friend, brother, son. We all have multiple roles and many demands on our time and energy. And then there's *you*. If I asked you which one of all these things you sacrificed, what would it be? Often it's our self. *I didn't go to the gym because I was too busy.*

I always try to make time to do the things that I know are part of me staying well. After I had depression I had to put my life back together again. I never wanted to feel like that again, and slowly I learned what it takes to stay well. It's a combination of things. It's about spending time with the people I love – like the evening meal that I've already written about. It's about being physically fit. It's about learning new things. It's about noticing the little things that bring me pleasure, so that they don't just pass me by but become part of my conscious experience – that cup of coffee; the feeling of hot water on my back in the shower. And it's also about the work

I do around depression awareness and mental health: I share my story and it helps people, and I've had more satisfaction from that than I had from being an All Black.

I have to do these things if I want to be well. It takes real determination. I often say to my wife, 'I'm selfish. I'm selfish because I need to be. And it makes me a better person.'

In being conscientious about these things – insisting that my wellness is everyday – I hope that I'm modelling good things for my kids. I hope they'll know how to live resiliently so they won't go through what I went through. I encourage them to take up interests that feed their mind and soul. Luca, for instance, has developed a passion for making things in wood. So we're really promoting that. If he's angry about something, we say, 'Well, go and make something!' That's what I'm trying to teach them. I said to Luca the other day, 'You've got such a gift with that guitar and singing. Go and do that when you're upset.'

'I don't feel like it.'

'Exactly. Go and try.'

This is a simple message that people find incredibly helpful. So many people say to me, 'I read *All Blacks Don't Cry* [or I went on the depression.org website] and I took your advice. I started running and now I'm addicted to it'; or 'I took up meditation'; or 'I learnt to play the ukulele.' There are 50 options; 1000 options. You don't know which one is right for you until you try.

I'm not perfect, not by any means. It takes willpower: it can be hard to find the time, but you've just got to. And it also takes self-forgiveness: if you let it slide for a few days, don't beat yourself up – but do get back into it. Make sure your kids know this. Encourage, support, prod them into finding things that work for them; but also teach them and model self-forgiveness when they find it hard to do these things.

If I'm chasing my tail at work, I let myself go physically. I like to get to the swimming pool or the gym each day – but maybe I don't go for four or five days.

I've still got the all-or-nothing tendencies I wrote about in *All Blacks Don't Cry* – I can't eat four chips, I eat the packet; I can't drink two glasses of wine, I drink the bottle. I really need to change that for my wellbeing and personal control. Every age has its phase, and I just can't live like I used to and expect to keep the same health.

I'm trying a few things and I'm working really hard on finding some balance. I've been doing the Fast Diet, and it's working well with my psychology. I fast two days a week – but the fun comes on the other days when I can eat and drink what I want. With my extremist nature it suits me, and I've lost a good amount of weight.

It wouldn't suit everyone. I reckon there's a market there somewhere: *the perfect diet for your psychology*. But that's the thing about wellness – you have to find what works and what fits and is meaningful for you.

Living to 100. I sometimes think we work the wrong way round when we think about our health. We should say, 'I want to live to 100 – now, what's the best way of achieving that?'

- Wellness is about finding and doing the things that make you feel good. Encourage and support your young person to find out what these are for them.
- Wellness is everyday.

66.
The little things you do each day

Flora: Lots of people think of your health as physical health, and it's really not. Wellbeing is physical, spiritual, mental and social.

JK: A big part of mental health is making sure you have time for yourself, time to do the things that relax you.

I'm an active relaxer. I don't like the TV, but I love to read books. I love to cook, I love to play my guitar, I love to swim and surf. These things all take me away from daily stresses, shift my thinking and open up some space in my mind. I don't talk about these things as 'goals' – I say they're emotions. Comfort. Peace. Warmth. Relaxation. The satisfaction of achievement.

Wellness for me is a living, breathing thing.

If you start setting goals for wellness you start putting pressure on yourself: *I've got to play the guitar today, and if I don't I'm not going to be well.* So I think of those things in terms of the feelings they give me. And that is wellness. There are things you need to do every day that feed your wellness, and chances are they'll be different to my things. A lot of people take up running, or meditation, or woodwork. Whatever feeds your soul. They do it for the feeling they get while they're doing it, or for the feeling they get when they've done it.

Elliot: What makes us happy? As a society over the past 60 years we've become wealthier, with greater access to consumer goods than any generation in the past. Yet mental illness – the biggest predictor of unhappiness – has also grown.

There seem to be three factors associated with happiness. First, people likely have a biological 'set point' which, like a thermostat, sets their happiness to a particular level; then there are objective circumstances; and finally, there are intentional behaviours and ways of thinking.

Fortunately, with regard to circumstances, income (beyond a certain basic level) does not seem to correlate with happiness. The really good news, though, is that the third factor – what you choose to do and how you think – has a substantial contribution and is within your control.

The New Zealand Mental Health Foundation is promoting the Five Ways to Wellbeing – a set of five evidence-based actions that you can choose to do that can improve wellbeing in everyday life. They are based on a large amount of research connecting them to wellbeing – and yet they aren't that hard: they are within everybody's reach. They are:

- Connect
- Give
- Take notice
- Keep learning
- Be active.

While a lot of the research was initially based on people aged 16 and up, internationally it has been found to apply to younger people as well – although with one slight change: creativity and play were additional actions associated with wellbeing. Brainstorm with your young person ways that they can increase their involvement in these areas.

As you can see, these fit beautifully with what JK figured out for himself about what works and what keeps him well. Wellness is about body and mind; it's about the little things you do each day.

Jacob: I skateboard a lot. I love skateboarding, and often, if I'm feeling stressed or low or want to chill out, I'll go skateboarding. Or I'll channel emotions into playing music. I wrote a lot of songs and played my instruments in my bedroom.

I read a lot of Buddhist kind of texts. That kind of general view that life is really beautiful and good, it really speaks to me. I wouldn't even say I hold Buddhist views, it's just a beautiful way of looking at life. One counsellor encouraged me to try meditation and I do that at times, although not as regularly as I should.

Olivia: Music. It helps you escape; it takes you somewhere else for a while. The lyrics of what you're listening to can change the way you're thinking.

JK: For me, it's not just the music – it's the moment. Music creates the moment. The more you do it and go to the music, your body and mind know that you're going to get some sort of relief from your moment. It's as if, through doing these things you love, you are creating pathways to wellbeing.

Olivia: Exercise.

Sophie: Taking a nap.

- Wellness is about body and mind. It's about the little things you do each day.
- The things we do and the way we think have a big impact on our level of happiness.
- The Five Ways to Wellbeing is a set of five simple actions that can improve wellbeing in everyday life. They are: Connect, Give, Take notice, Keep learning, Be active.

67.
Surfing the moment

JK: Surfing is one of my favourite pastimes. It works on at least four levels for me: my fitness, my spirituality, it's something I'm still learning – and my kids are into it. Those things are really important for me in my wellness, and I can do them all in one surfing session.

I'm trying to take my surfing back to old-school, 1960s-style surfing, using a longboard, walking the board or hanging ten. Surfing with a lot more style, and I'm just trying to improve. Mostly, it's about taking my mind to another place – drifting in the middle of the ocean, just waiting, enjoying the moment.

Enjoying the moment is a skill you have to work on a bit; you need to wash away some of the stress before you can truly 'enjoy the moment'. Often I'll be like a bee in a bonnet when I first get out there – I've got all this nervous energy and I rush into the first few waves. I'm the city boy who's been rushing around, rushed to the beach to have a surf, and the first 20 minutes are still at a million miles an hour. But then I start calming into the moment: I become a bit more Zen-like. Then I think, *what am I doing? I'm never going to be world champ . . . I should slow down and enjoy myself.* And then I begin to forget about stuff and enjoy the moment.

It's very hard to enjoy the moment when you're stressed or carrying stuff with you, and I find that surfing washes that away a wee bit.

I really enjoy the sea. It gives me peace. When I'm driving along beside it in the mornings I'll stop the car sometimes and look at it, and it makes me feel peaceful. I just take it in and enjoy it for what it is. I try not to take it for granted.

Swimming is another water-based activity that I love. When I'm in a good routine I'll go to the pool, usually early in the morning. I swim up and down – I'll do two, maybe three kilometres – and I get into a rhythm that's a bit meditational. I get in a zone and I can think about stuff in a really relaxed way. That's quite different from what happens in my mind when I'm surfing. With swimming, I can actually problem-solve. No one can disturb me, no one can talk to me, no one stops me.

68.
Learning to ask for help

Hannah: What I got out of the eating disorder experience was an awareness of my own anxiety that I didn't previously have, so I can now recognise it and do something about it. And I now know that it's OK to ask for help.

That's been huge for me, because I do work every day to stay well, and I wouldn't be able to do that without my exceptionally strong support network, especially my parents. I'm living away from home now, at university in a different city, and I've had to learn to cut myself some slack. Be kind to myself. My expectations . . . the goalposts have shifted definitely, permanently, as a result of my experience – and not in a bad way. I think I'm more productive for that. The other thing is that the new friends I've met at uni and my flatmates – I wasn't planning it, but I ended up telling people, giving them a brief history of my mental health or whatever. That's really important because I know that if they noticed me deteriorating in any way, eating or anxiety, they would text Mum or Dad. They would do something.

In less healthy moments, I wish I hadn't told them, but that's why it's so important – because it's that extra barrier to relapse.

If I'm having an anxious moment I remove myself from the situation and just take five to 10 minutes to totally regroup. One of the biggest markers for my anxiety is my thinking just gets so fuzzy and weird, completely irrational, so if I notice that and take a few minutes and think things through logically, or think about what's happened and then go back to the situation I was in – which is affirming in itself that I've managed to go back out there – that's something that helps.

I have some anti-anxiety medication that I've been prescribed. I've probably taken about two pills in the past year, but it's helpful to know it's there.

I've learnt to ask for help. I've learnt to externalise. I can ring up Mum and Dad and say, 'Help.'

Sometimes it's just a comment to friends: 'I'm not feeling great this week.' I'm lucky that my friends know what I mean. They look out for me a bit more. Other times, it's been 'Dad, get on the plane right now, I need help.' That's more direct. I find it easier to ask for help from someone who I know will understand.

It's been hard for me. One of the reasons Mum and Dad never delved deeper at the beginning is that I've always made a huge effort to present as capable and together and I know what I'm doing and I'm fine and all that sort of stuff. So it's hard to be the one asking for help. But I know I wouldn't be well right now if 20 times in the past year I hadn't asked for help.

Kirsty: Hannah makes a really important point – a key part of staying well is being able to recognise when things are becoming stressful, and then accepting the support needed to get through. Encourage your young person to plan ahead of time who they might approach for support. Who are the people they would go to if things became difficult? Brainstorm as many options as possible, encouraging your young person to think about the types of support that different people offer. Write the names and contact details down, or store them in your young person's phone so that they're available when needed.

69.
Building confidence and staying well

JK: The biggest effect depression had on me was that it took away my confidence in what I was great at. I worked hard on – and continue to work hard on – my mental wellness and rewiring my brain, and I think I'm really competent at that now; but I didn't really work towards rebuilding my confidence about my sport. Perhaps if I'd been more open about the effect it had had on me . . . But I also think there's a lot more known now about how to manage the pressures of sport at the professional level.

Lyndy Matthews (psychiatrist): Depression shatters your confidence. When you're physically ill you use your mind to cope with the illness, but if you've got an illness of the mind you can't use your mind to help you cope, and that can have long-term effects on your confidence. I see that particularly in the young people I treat, because they're finding their feet in terms of their confidence and identity anyway.

So you might have a kid who, because there wasn't an early diagnosis, had two years of depressed mood and depressed brain function. That kid will feel that their brain isn't working properly, that their thinking isn't sharp. Even once the depression has past, they might still have lost their knack and their confidence – so the problem is both psychological and biological.

We deal with it by identifying the problem and talking about it. I say: 'This is about your confidence. This is not about your brain not working. Your brain is working again now. This is just

something that might take a little time – it's like a muscle that you have to exercise.'

Jacob: Because of my depression and my drug-taking, I left school without any qualifications. I'm 20 now, drug-free and I'm doing a foundation course at a polytech.

Being in a learning situation after so long is great in every way! I do not struggle with the material we are learning, only with the ability to manage myself and my time properly. We all know I have issues with my memory and concentration, although I feel like it's getting better. But I'm still not a very confident person. There's a lot of self-doubt – socially, in my opinions, and where I stand.

I'm really busy, though. I'm in a band and I'm learning a new sport. I'm reading lots and loving that. I try and eat well. And I like meditating, although I don't always get around to it. I'm happier than I've been for years, which is partly why I was happy to contribute to this book. I think I'm better at recognising the signs in myself. I haven't slipped into a deep dark hole of depression for about 18 months. If I'm feeling low I'm good at recognising it, and the next day I can wake up feeling OK, and it's just that day, that moment.

- Depression takes away your self-confidence.
- Even once the depression has passed, it can take time to rebuild clarity of thinking, memory and confidence.

70.
Becoming mindful

JK: I'm interested in the effect of meditation and prayer on recovery and wellbeing.

I believe there's a god but I don't know whether he's the Catholic god, or the Anglican god, or Allah. I don't pray. Instead, for me, I get that 'god' feeling through being at peace with myself – taking time to read, to play guitar. When it comes to spirituality I think it's how you live, in the sense of living a good life. For me, that's about being a good dad, being a good person, trying to be a good influence on the people around me, giving back to the community.

As I said in *All Blacks Don't Cry*, a wise priest, talking to me about my beliefs, asked me if I had love in my life. 'Yes,' I replied. 'Well,' he said, 'God is love.' So for me, that's what it's all about. Feeling the love. Living a good life. That's my soul food.

Elliot: In terms of psychological science and the psychological treatment of depression, a relevant development is the adoption of an aspect of Buddhist meditation practice – mindfulness – into cognitive behaviour therapy.

Mindfulness can be thought of as a non-judgmental, in-the-moment awareness of the thoughts, feelings and physical sensations we experience. Its application in CBT involves teaching clients the practice of mindfulness to help them combat the natural tendency in depression to ruminate. Rumination is the constant preoccupation with distress that is one of the hallmarks of the illness. Rumination and worry can escalate very quickly in depression, and bring about rapid, severe and sustained drops in mood.

Mindfulness enables clients to break that escalating process by identifying their thoughts and feelings as *just* thoughts and feelings, and letting them go. Mindfulness-based cognitive therapy is a proven treatment with adults that was developed to help people who had previous experience of depression to stay well. This is very significant because of the episodic nature of depression and the increasing risk of further episodes with each episode experienced.

The same evidence base has yet to be established with adolescents, but there is considerable research being undertaken on teaching mindfulness to depressed teens, and also to children generally in schools, to enhance their ability to manage their emotions.

JK: I did try meditation, but found I was unable to sit still. However, I think that through my activities like surfing and swimming and playing the guitar, I have developed my own way of becoming mindful and peaceful. One of the things I can do now is to let thoughts go. They still come into my head, but then they float up a chimney – this is what I imagine – and out and away.

Elliot: JK's chimney is a very useful image. Another way to think about it is to imagine you're standing in a room and thoughts and feelings are coming in and going out – like guests passing through, in other words. But when you're depressed and anxious, the thoughts and feelings come in and don't leave, so that eventually you are in the room with a crowd of black thoughts and the doors and windows are closed.

Research is ongoing into the relationship between spirituality and wellbeing. This is obviously a very complex area, but there is some evidence that people who use spiritual coping methods such as meditation, prayer and attendance at church may experience greater wellbeing and more positive health outcomes. Alongside possible spiritual explanations, psychological accounts for this might include the connections to a resilient social environment that belonging to a church might provide; along with the cultivation of hope, and the facilitation of forgiveness and letting go. Also, common to many faiths is a focus on 'virtues' such as courage, humanity and temperance, and these things have been identified as attributes associated with wellbeing within the field of positive psychology as well.

- There may be some wellbeing benefits associated with spirituality.
- The practice of mindfulness – an aspect of Eastern meditation traditions – is increasingly being incorporated into contemporary Western psychological treatments.

71. Wellness is dangerous

JK: So, wellness is everyday. The other thing I've learnt is: wellness is dangerous. You do all your wellness things and you start to feel great. You feel so good that you stop doing the things that have helped you get to that level, and that's when you can start to re-enter the danger zone.

It's important that you don't think you're cured forever. Don't ever take it for granted. You've got to keep revisiting your wellness – keep checking in with it. If you're getting bored with your routine, try something new. It's an ongoing journey. The worst thing you can do when you come through this illness is think you're well.

Kirsty: Adolescents are particularly good (or bad) at this. A positive relationship change – for instance, a new boyfriend or girlfriend – and all of a sudden the world is perfect again, and they don't need to bother with working on being well or worrying about all that stuff or seeing the therapist again. However, we would always recommend at least one final session or one sit-down with the young person, the parent or a mentor, where you celebrate the person feeling well and go through the strategies we mentioned earlier – recognising what it would look like if it popped up again, and what the young person needs to do if it does. Have this written down on a piece of paper! They may not read or need it then because 'life is perfect', but they have it to go back to when life throws the next curveball.

JK: I'm still searching for the perfect balance in my life. With my obsessive, all-or-nothing nature, that's a tough thing to achieve. But what I have achieved is a sense of self-acceptance: I've accepted I'm like that, so I don't beat myself up or negative self-talk myself. I just get back on the wagon and on I go.

It's a journey. You never stop growing. I want to be incredibly well – physically, mentally, spiritually, emotionally – so I've got to keep working on it. I hope I'll still be saying the same thing at one hundred.

PART NINE
Stand By Me

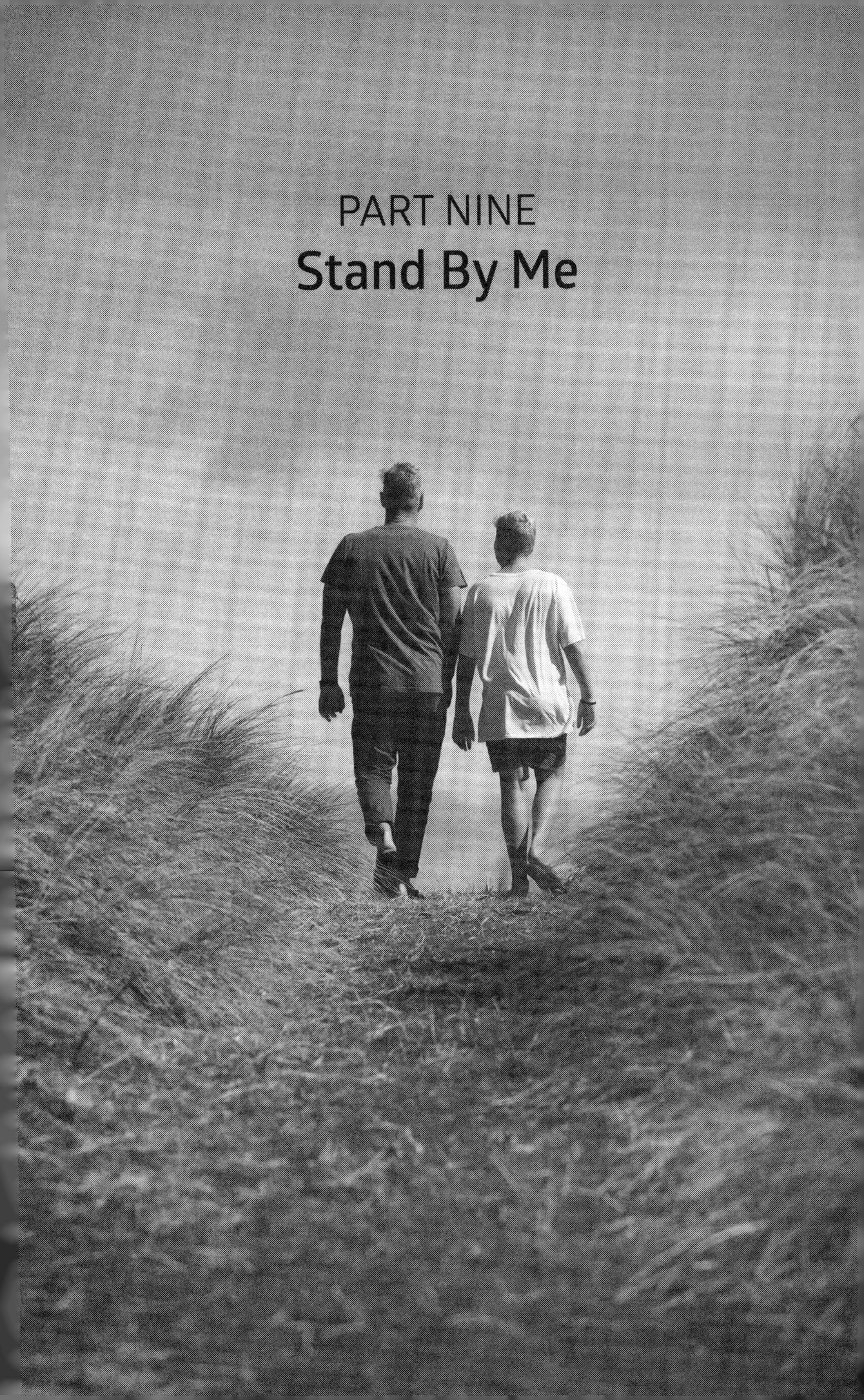

72.
Stand by me

JK: One of the best things I've done was meeting with the two classrooms of Auckland secondary-school students. It made me a better parent straight away, just sitting and listening to them; and for me that's what 'stand by me' is now: I need to listen a lot more to my kids, I need to emphasise to them that I am there, but I'm not trying to verbally parent them all the time. I'm giving them a little bit more freedom.

The kids at Mt Albert Grammar gave me some crucial information. They want their parents to ask them how they are, but they want their parents to understand that they aren't always ready to talk just yet. That doesn't mean they don't *want* to talk; it might just mean they haven't sorted things out in their own mind yet, or that they're gathering their courage. But they do want their parents to come back later and ask again.

They want their parents to be parents. They don't want us to say the latest slang – I thought I was cool saying 'Up-G', but it turns out I was just being embarrassing. They don't want us to lecture, or to go on and on about things: 'Don't give us the PowerPoint presentation,' as one girl said. They want us to listen, not leap in with our own judgments.

I was amazed that they want us to get to know their friends. Mostly – with some exceptions – they thought that if things were going badly for them, it would be OK for parents to check in with their friends.

They really like it when we notice that things are stressful for them, and step in to carry the load in practical ways – maybe cooking a nice dinner, or making their bed for them.

So what does 'Stand by me' look like? It's not 'Stand by me and talk all the time.' It's not lecturing. It's just, 'Be there when I need you.'

When we started doing this book I had a whole lot of questions I needed answering. Now I know that some questions can't be answered – for instance, what is the exact right thing to do and say when your child is in trouble? But I do understand how I can stand by my children a lot better.

I took Luca out to the beach when we were doing the photo-shoot for the book's cover, and afterwards a woman came up to me. Her son had been in trouble with depression a few years previously and she'd asked me to talk to him, and she wanted to thank me. She told me he is now in really good shape. After we'd finished talking, Luca said to me, 'Gee, that must feel very special, Dad, when that happens.'

'Yeah,' I said, 'it's really special.'

Then he said, 'Why? Why do they thank you so much?' And I realised that, because he's just a kid, he really had no idea about my depression and the whole background to the public awareness campaign. So I took the opportunity: I told him that what had happened to me was really scary. I said, 'If you ever feel anything like that, mate, I'm here. Come and see me and we'll talk about it and you'll be fine. Don't ever be afraid to reach out and get help.' It was a chance to make a couple of key points.

It was a 'stand by me' moment. I didn't want to go into it too much. I didn't want to scare him, but I knew he would have been thinking, *what if that happens to me?*

So now I understand: those moments need to come from them, but they happen because you're standing by them, listening for those moments. So I've changed a wee bit. I'm listening for those moments.

I'm not trying to preach to them. I guess you could say I'm actively listening – listening to catch what's lying behind the things they say.

73.
Reach out

Kirsty: We use words like 'protective factors'. What makes it so that, even though tough things are going on in your life, you're OK?

Sophie: People to lean on. Because most of the things you're feeling, to some degree the people around you are feeling as well. If you're insecure about something, the chances are one of your other friends is going to be feeling insecure as well.

Ellen: I think it's support. I reckon that even if all these things are going really horribly but you have support, you'll be able to get through it. But if you don't have support, you're just screwed.

JK: Getting support can make all the difference to someone when they're down. I feel really bad for kids who feel they have no one – it's hard to reach out, especially when you're depressed. Hayley didn't feel she had anyone to talk to, but now she reckons it could have made a difference, and she recommends that anyone who is being bullied and feeling lonely reaches out to someone – as long as that person understands their role is support. Support isn't necessarily about taking over, or getting really bossy – it can just be listening and reflecting: 'Yeah, that sounds really hard. You're doing really well. I'm here for you when you need to talk or if you need a shoulder to cry on.' The thing that strikes me when I hear the stories of the kids in this book is that, having been through such tough times themselves, they all want to help and support others.

Helene: Knowing there are people who will stick by you and give you their love is crucial. My family has been so important for me – to know that, no matter what, they'll always be there. If I didn't have that I don't know where I'd be.

I never completely lost hope, and that was the thing that always kept me together. I could look beyond and imagine things would get better, and that was probably because I was so supported. I felt at times like I'd trapped myself in a situation, and I was basically struggling to keep my head above water. I felt trapped because you're not supposed to give up or quit – but once I realised that actually you can walk away from something that's just not good for you and it's not going to be the end of the world, there was a relief, and a bit of space. I understand that there are some environments or conditions that aren't good for me and I'm OK with that.

Jacob: Mum, my family, they were incredibly helpful even when I didn't see it. I didn't think they understood, but I'm sure they totally did. That's that family thing, though, and it can get quite conflicted.

I have a much older sister I'm close to, and she was someone I reached out to if I wanted to relax and just feel safe. If your parents are telling you this one thing and you don't believe it or you refuse to believe it, and you go off and speak to someone like my sister, she might say the same thing, and you go, 'Oh yeah, OK, OK.'

My uncle. I remember him taking me out to the movies with his girlfriend and, though I was very conscious of it being because I'd had this episode and it was kind of awkward and we didn't talk about it, it was still really nice to have that gesture shown.

I guess what was nice and helpful was where you might be really down and a hug is really nice. And there's the constructive feedback to try and encourage me.

Friends – I let a lot go through those years. I had a close friend who was very understanding when I was going through my panic attacks. If I was having one at school she'd take me out of class or wherever. When I went missing one time the police rang some of my mates, and that's how they found out I'd tried to kill myself. One mate was really cool about it. I remember him saying, 'You can't do that, eh bro! You can't! Life's good,' kind of stuff, and I remember really appreciating it.

Levi: The most important thing that I've found is support. When you say 'support' to me I just think of someone behind me, but then I think about it more and I realise it's even more than that: it's consistency, courage and faith. It's about, when you get to the point where you think, *I can't do this no more*, then that support is still there, not giving up on you.

I think the main thing is just not to give up on someone you are helping. If Matt had given up on me I'd be in jail right now. I would not be who I am, I would not know who I am. But because of Matt's strength to not give up on me, that support has got me to where I am today: and today I'm a youth worker, I'm a security guard, a musician, a singer-songwriter; to express my feelings I write music, I go to church, I sing at church, and I serve my community. That's a lot coming from zero. And my favourite job – I wouldn't say it's a job, but it's a mission – is serving my community. It is helping those who need that support, and that's always the highlight of my day.

A lot of kids don't have families to support them. But the issues are the same – they need someone to be their friend and not give up on them.

Hayley: By the end of Year 10 I was seeing more of my mum, and eventually I went to live with her. I told her what was happening and she helped me move schools. But by that stage my anxiety had got so bad that I had this constant scared feeling – a feeling that, at any moment, something really, really bad might happen. I couldn't concentrate in class, and I was breaking down every morning before school, faking sick, crying. I ended up going to school less and less until they kicked me out, really. I'd just turned sixteen.

I'd started coming down to ZEAL, first just to listen to bands, and I began to get to know the other volunteers. One of the girls needed someone to help her do the café at a show, and I said I'd help. I felt a connection there. It was a new group of friends who weren't like the high-school kids.

Once I left school the anxiety started to go away: I was not so stressed out. I got more involved at ZEAL. Now I go there every day. I volunteer, and I work in the café. It's a safe place and I'm getting better. It's a really supportive, friendly environment. I'm in a place where I belong.

Because of their support, I'm learning to trust people. I'm learning how to deal with the fears that I still have. In the past week it's happened that I've had those thoughts – *they don't really like me* – and I can say to myself, *actually, if they didn't like me I'd know. They wouldn't be as close as they are. They wouldn't hang out with me.*

I don't know what I want to do in the future, but at the moment I'm just really happy doing what I'm doing, and not feeling sick from stress.

My experiences have definitely changed me. But if I had a choice I would still have gone through it, because even though it felt so bad I'm such a better person now from it. I understand more. I understand people's feelings more, and I'm sensitive to that. And with other people getting picked on, I know what it's like, and I can help them.

Amitai: My fresh start came when I told my mother I was gay. I was scared for myself because the negative talk was becoming too intense. I was becoming physically sick and wanting to take my life on a regular basis. When it came to telling my mother, I was in such a state I was hyperventilating and couldn't speak. She tried her best to figure out what was going wrong, and as she cycled through her greatest fears of what I could be so upset about, she asked, 'Son, are you gay?' I felt the words burn in my mouth: 'Mum, I'm gay' – but at the same time I felt an incredible weight lift from my heart. My fear subsided and I could breathe again. I knew that as long as the people I cared about loved and accepted me, things were going to be better. I didn't have to face things alone.

Now I have a very supportive boss and a group of friends who are so important to keeping me mentally well. I've accepted that I can't be strong 100 percent of the time, and actually that's OK.

- Support isn't necessarily about taking over, or getting really bossy – it can just be listening and reflecting.
- Support is about consistency, courage and faith.
- Support is about being in a place where you belong.
- Support is having people who will go in to bat for you.
- Support is people accepting and loving who you are.

74.
Share the load

Matt (Levi's new dad): I met Levi when I was taking a boxing class at ZEAL. He came into the youth centre and decided to join the boxing programme. Boxing attracts the young guys who've had it rough; it's a great outlet for them, and they probably crave a little bit of discipline and order. So Levi was 15 or 16 when I first met him. I saw in him what I see in a lot of young people – the two sides. The side he puts forward in public: quite cocky, talented, abrasive, probably masking his wariness and insecurity about coming into a new environment. But I also saw a different side, a softer side, and I saw him looking to connect in some way, but also a bit fearful of doing that, about being vulnerable. It takes a leap of faith to be vulnerable, and he wrestled with that a little bit.

At that stage it's really important for me to remain constant and be the person who's willing to take the first step in vulnerability. A lot of it is about consistency. Even the practical things, like making sure that the boxing is always on – that one week it wouldn't be cancelled – because those young guys, they'll take that personally. *See, someone else let me down.* They won't come back.

So it's the practical things; and the little things, like genuinely asking how he is after the boxing, letting him know quite clearly that I care about him. Not expecting anything back. Just leave it at that, and 'I'll see you next week.' So they know they can trust you. And not putting up with any shit. It's the same as any dad would with kids – it's teaching them how to treat people as well. So slowly they learn that it's OK, and they see me take steps of vulnerability and slowly they do as well, and Levi definitely did that.

Levi had missed out on a lot in his life, but I never really felt I could fill the gap. That was never an intention. It's important to not come with an expectation of change. I think that's where a lot of people who help others can get caught up in these expectations of change for a young person, so when the young person doesn't meet those expectations the whole relationship breaks down.

Through circumstances and events, Levi just genuinely became like a son to me and I took on a bit of a fathering role, so it was organic in that way. It just became normal for me to care for him and love him. It was less about wanting to change this guy. It was more about: *he needs a place to live and so – of course. I love him. I don't want him living under a bridge or in a boys' home.*

Sometimes he'd be making steps towards change, but then his old life would catch up with him and he'd disappear for a week or so, and I'd get a phone call at three in the morning with him in tears going, 'Sorry, I let you down,' so I'd pick him up and bring him home.

I wouldn't be angry, but I'd definitely be disappointed. I think that was really important, because we would rob young people if we didn't get disappointed or have human reactions to things. And he said later that when he did do something silly, what brought him home was knowing that he'd let me down.

Levi had experienced a lot of rejection and inconsistency. He needed never to doubt that he could come back to our house, and that probably goes back to the expectation thing: I'm not doing this because he's going to become an angel, but because I care about him. And even the letting me down – I'd just get really worried about him. And I do have expectations of him now as a father, but those expectations are never a barrier. It's like, *I'm holding you to account*, rather than, *this is a make or break kind of thing*. My love for him is unconditional.

Levi just became part of the family. And it's really important for my children, too. People would say, 'What about your kids? How well do you really know this guy? What if he hurt your kids?' But a big thing for us with our biological kids is that they grow up to be compassionate. You can't learn that in a book. My daughter gave up her room for Levi. We're so proud of her for that. She felt good about herself, and she knew that she was making a difference.

When Levi's 'black dog' comes, I just be with him. It's just going, 'That's awful,' and connecting with that brokenness and just sitting with it. And there's something about that, about sharing suffering. Saying: 'What you're saying is painful. I'm feeling that pain, and let's feel it together.' And I think for someone who's in that pain, to be able to share that suffering with someone else, it's the biggest gift – and any caregiver can do that. It's probably a bit unnatural, because I know that with my own kids, when they hurt themselves, I just want to fix it; but I think it's really important with mental health to just sit there and suffer alongside.

Maybe it's because part of the pain of depression is it's so isolating, and what you want, when you're feeling that really heavy sadness, is just to crawl under a bed and be alone. But to have someone crawl under that bed with you, then at least you're not in there alone. At that really hard moment, it's not about bringing them out, but it's just sitting through it and maybe it shares the load spiritually a bit.

75.
Through the choppy waters

Catherine (Sean's mum): *Stand By Me* – what a great title for this book.

Tragically, some people with depression do kill themselves; and there were times when Sean's doctor would have concerns and restrict his medication, or check on him to see if she thought he was safe. But Sean wrote Geoff and me this letter – a letter I keep in my wallet at all times – and because it's written down in black and white I believe him when he says he wouldn't kill himself. He is very deep-thinking and mindful of what we've been through during those times when we've stood by him.

> Dearest Ma and Pa,
> Although I have tough times a lot, one thing I want you to know is that I will never give up. I could never do that to you. The pain I feel is nothing compared to the pain that I would cause you and everyone around me if I was to take an easy way out. I could never put you through that. At the moment I can't see the light at the end of the tunnel but I believe there is one because you both do. If I could grow to be a small fraction of the caring, loving and beautiful people that you both are then it's worth the struggle. I'll never forget how much you've done for me and I'll always be appreciative of that. I love you more than anything, even my music.
> Love, Sean

I don't see the lengths we've gone to for Sean as a sacrifice. I just see it as part of our journey. When I pushed that child out I didn't imagine for one moment that this was going to be our journey, but it *is* our journey. We might want to say *why us*? But equally we can say *why not*? Not that I'm saying we're overjoyed it's all happened, but it has and – as we all know . . . shit happens! You can't change any of that. And it's what you do with your experience that's the most important thing. You can't keep saying, *woe is me*. You have to be proactive. You have to be there for your children. Parenting is forever. You're in for the long haul. It's not just for the good times, it's for all time. So we're in it, aren't we? Till the very end.

We've stuck by Sean like glue. I'm sure that a lot of people have thought we've been far too soft and we needed to practise the old-fashioned 'tough love' thing. I think that's all very well and good when you're dealing with a run-of-the-mill adolescent, but when depression is put into the mix everything changes.

Sean's had a couple of friends who have had similar issues but haven't had the same support. He's told us he knows he's extremely lucky to have had us. But I don't consider him to be 'lucky'. Luck's got nothing to do with it. It's every child's right to be loved and supported unconditionally.

There's no doubt about it, living with someone who is depressed is just the hardest journey, and when that someone is your child, it's the pits. But as I've said, the 'black dog' has been in our life for a reason and we have to embrace it for what it is and deal with it. Take the good stuff from all the bad and work with it in a positive way. That's exactly what JK's done.

I work at a school in a musical capacity. A little while ago my friend and I taught the school a Maori proverb set to music – *He moana pukepuke e ekingia e te waka* – which means 'Your boat will get through these choppy waters'. In other words, persevere and never give up. Every time I played it I'd think of Sean and say to myself, *we are going to get through these choppy waters!* And here we are, six years on . . . and our boat is turning towards the shore.

76.
The armour of vulnerability

JK: The title of this book, *Stand By Me*, is really important to me. When I'm stressed or under pressure or not feeling bulletproof, I go back to the people I love the most. I need them around me. That's my comfort zone. We all need someone to 'stand by me', and that's about letting our guards down, being vulnerable and open, and asking for or accepting help.

Vulnerability is one of the most important characteristics in our relationships. It's about having the courage to be honest, open, no pretences. Our kids are much more likely to let us stand by them if we show them our vulnerable side, too.

It's 10 years now since I first went on TV to talk about my experience of depression, becoming part of the Ministry of Health's campaign to destigmatise mental illness. I could never have dreamed, back at the beginning, how that campaign would change my life. Over those years I've met so many New Zealanders, all sorts of people, from all walks of life – hundreds, thousands of people – who have shared their stories with me. They come up to me in the street, in the supermarket, in airport waiting lounges, at events, and they tell me what's going on in their lives. They show me their vulnerability. It's a great gift. They do that because I've been vulnerable on those TV ads for the past 10 years, and so people trust me. They're vulnerable to me and I'm vulnerable back, and they trust me with that and I trust them straight back. It's an amazing human connection.

As a family, Fiorella, Niko, Luca and I do lots of things together – we eat the evening meal together, go to social events together. I take my boys surfing; I talk to my daughter on Skype as often as possible. We lounge around on the sofa on Sunday afternoons and watch TV and sleep. We get out and toss the ball around. But you know what our important emotional glue is? Vulnerability.

When was the last time you told your family you were scared? I think as parents we're scared of vulnerability. We think, *we're the parents*: we need to be in control at all times; we need to look like we know what we're doing. But I try to be as vulnerable as I can, and that means: take down your defences, your pretences, and show the people you love who you really are. I don't try and be tough at home.

Layla (Christie's mum): Being very open and telling people what was going on was how we found our strength and got our support. Everyone at work knew, so I didn't feel I had to maintain this bravado and this exterior of having everything in control. If I dissolved in tears at work everyone knew why. I guess it came back to knowing this is an illness. It's not something Christie chose to have happen, it's not something I caused.

I went and talked to her class at school. I decided right from the beginning, we're not going to be ashamed of this. It's an illness, a mental illness, triggered by mental imbalance.

So being really open took one pressure away. People knew I was having a difficult time, friends knew, so there was no extra expectation or pressure, and people would offer to help. That was really important. Not being ashamed that your child has got a mental illness is really, really vital, because you can't help them if you're feeling that, or if you're preoccupied by thinking that in some ways you're less than whole as a person.

Helene: It might have helped if I had realised that anxiety is an illness and not a personality fault. In my mind it was always my fault. Discovering that other people have similar feelings was the first thing that made me feel better. When people described feelings and thoughts that were exactly like mine, it was . . . Well, it still makes me cry today. And when I tell people what's happened to me, then it's much more likely that they'll share their experiences – and that also helps my awareness that other people go through it, too.

I told some of my close friends about it soon after the event. Some of them were a bit surprised. No one had a negative reaction. Some of them couldn't relate and others could. Sometimes, the people I thought might not understand were the ones who understood best of all. I was amazed one day to get a phone call from a guy I'd known at school – he was not a talker at all, quite a classic Kiwi guy in that man-of-few-words way, and I'd often wondered what was going on under there. Anyway, he said he wanted to have a chat with me. He said: 'I think I've been depressed for 15 years.'

When you are open about your experiences it frees people to be more open about their own. It's amazing how people respond. My boss at work was very open with us about his daughter having a mental illness, and in doing so he showed a warmer and more vulnerable side to himself that hadn't been so visible before. It's all part of the human experience.

JK: When I'm at home with my family, I make myself vulnerable and honest around whatever my pressure points are at that time. I'm not one of these people who say, 'Let's send the kids to bed so we can talk.' Ninety percent of the time I'll discuss anything with the kids. If I show vulnerability, then they'll learn to show it. If I show them who I really am, they'll show me who they really are.

If I've got a big game coming up and I'm worried about how my team is doing, I'll tell my family about it. I'll say, 'We're not where we need to be and I'm worried about it.' Their first reaction is always protection of me: 'It's up to the players; you're working really hard . . .' But my reaction is to say to them: 'Yeah, but what am I missing?' I say that because that's what keeps *me* awake at night – *What am I missing? How can I do better?* – and so I share it with them. They give me some really good answers. Kids often have a very simple solution. And it means they're involved in my life and they see me as a real person.

Because I'm vulnerable with my kids, they can be vulnerable back at me. Vulnerability paves the way to honest interactions.

When we started working on this book, my biggest fear was that I didn't have the skills to parent my kids through their tough times. I had so many questions, most of them starting with 'What do I do when . . .?' I needed answers, and I thought those answers were going to be like a toolkit – a bag of custom-built tools: 'When this happens, use this tool . . .' If only!

Doing this book has been a real journey for me. I've let go of some of my ideas. Now I know there is not always – or even often – a 'correct' answer to any of life's difficulties. And I've also figured out that we can't rescue our kids from everything life will throw at them. But we can stand by them. We can listen to them carefully and without judgment. We can love the real child. We can keep our relationships with them open and honest.

When it comes to my experience of mental illness, I'm open with my kids. I don't make a big deal of it. If you talk about it as a big event, it becomes a big event. My whole idea is to break down stigma and make it normal: it's part of my life, and in that way it's just normal. I only talk about it if they ask, and then I just answer. I let it come naturally.

I'm hoping to give them the skills to manage their emotions and their lives so that won't happen to them. I hope I'm living resiliently and that I'm teaching them how to do that, too. *You're feeling a bit stressed? What's your out?* If I give them that, their mental health won't be an issue. Hoping!

Resources

This section provides website and book suggestions that give further information about some of the areas covered in this book. Online resources are now plentiful, and the great thing about these is that they can be easily updated as new resources are developed or new information becomes available. Sometimes, however, the large number of sites available can seem overwhelming and it's hard to pick out the useful information. We recommend the following when trying to negotiate the potential information overload on the web.

- Start with an organisation that has a known reputation for providing sound information – a medical or research institute, a government-funded agency, or a good reputation as a community or consumer organisation. Most websites will have an 'About us' section that can give you an idea of where the information on the site is coming from and how reliable it may be.
- Take some time to look for the different sections within the website – many websites will have a parent/caregiver section as well as a young person's section; they will likely have resource sections; and some may have sibling sections.
- Start with some of the general one-page information sheets to get an overview of an area, and then move to more specific issues that are of interest.
- Most sites will have a list of resources with recommendations of other sites or agencies. These are a great way to find

further more specific information or supports that suit your needs.

- If you find a website you like, they will often have other ways you can connect with them – for example, through Facebook, or an email list where you can keep updated about any new resources, connect with like-minded people, and receive tips and encouragement.

The websites noted below are all great starting points. Almost all of them have information sheets, videos of people talking about their experiences, and sections that assist with connecting with online and local resources. They contain information about managing mental health when things are tough, and most also have information about wellness and fostering resilience.

General Mental Health and Wellbeing

Websites

aacap.org
American Academy of Child and Adolescent Psychiatry. Under the 'Facts for Families' section it has one-page information sheets covering a wide range of mental health and wellbeing areas. (US)

au.reachout.com
Youth mental health and wellbeing website covering a large range of topics with fact sheets, stories, videos, guides and apps, and an online forum. (Australia)

biteback.org.au/things-to-do/
Youth website run by the Black Dog Institute, with ways to improve wellbeing and mental fitness. (Australia)

blackdoginstitute.org.au
Research institute with good resources on depression and mental health. (Australia)

commonground.org.nz
Website with information about youth mental health, including ways to start conversations in this area, actions to take, and opportunities for people to tell their stories. (NZ)

headspace.org.nz; headspace.org.au
Resources for youth, families and schools covering general mental health fact sheets, good links to other resources, and tips for wellbeing. (NZ, Australia)

mentalhealth.org.nz
The Mental Health Foundation website with an A to Z of resources, links to support services, a list of e-therapy options and resources, and a section on strategies to improve your wellbeing. (NZ)

rethink.org/carers-family-friends/brothers-and-sisters-siblings-network/youth-siblings-area
Mental health site with a comprehensive section for siblings of people with mental health and for carers of people with mental health concerns. (UK)

skylight.org.nz
Wide range of resources on grief, mental health and wellbeing for children, adolescents and adults. Includes information sheets, links to resources, resource packs, and individual and group counselling support in some areas. (NZ)

thebalancedmind.org
Networking and resource site for carers of young people with depression or bipolar disorder. (US)

urge.co.nz
Youth health website with resources on emotional wellbeing, alcohol, drugs and relationships, and a services directory that allows you to search for local support services under chosen categories. (NZ)

youthline.co.nz
Fact sheets for parents and youth, along with information regarding their face to face counselling support, text support, phone support and email parent support service. (NZ)

Books

Braaten, E.B. (2011). *How to Find Mental Health Care for Your Child.* Washington: American Psychological Association

Carr-Gregg. M. (2010). *When to Really Worry: Mental health problems in teenagers and what to do about them.* Victoria: Penguin

Depression and Anxiety

Websites

depression.org.nz/waythrough/self+help
myjournal.depression.org.nz
Information on depression and wellness for older adolescents and adults. Includes an online self-help programme (The Journal), with a focus on strategies and techniques to promote wellness and help you get through mild to moderate depression. (NZ)

moodgym.anu.edu.au/moodgym
Free online interactive cognitive behaviour therapy programme with modules designed to address areas associated with low mood. (Australia)

parentingstrategies.net
Website that provides a comprehensive PDF covering ways to parent to prevent or reduce the impact of depression or anxiety on young people. (Australia)

smilingmind.com.au
Website and free app that facilitates use of mindfulness meditation to improve wellbeing. (Australia)

sparx.org.nz
Free online e-therapy tool using an avatar-based computer game. Based on cognitive behaviour therapy, it helps young people learn skills to deal with feeling down, depressed or anxious. (NZ)

thelowdown.co.nz
Interactive website for young people, with a self-test for depression, fact sheets, videos of people who have experience of depression, and text, phone and email support. (NZ)

worrywisekids.org
Website created by Tamar Chansky, with information and strategies for parents and young people with anxiety. (US)

youthbeyondblue.com
beyondblue.org.au/resources/family-and-friends/parents-and-guardians
Comprehensive information on depression and anxiety, including warning signs and options for seeking help, helping others and getting well. (Australia)

Books

Chansky, T. (2004). *Freeing Your Child from Anxiety.* New York, NY: Three Rivers Press

Fassler, D.G. & L.S. Dumas (1997). *Help Me, I'm Sad: Recognizing, treating and preventing childhood and adolescent depression.* New York: Penguin

Johnstone, M. (2005). *I had a Black Dog.* Australia: Pan Macmillan

Johnstone, M. & Johnstone, A. (2008). *Living with the Black Dog.* Australia: Pan Macmillan

Tompkins, M.A. & K.A. Martinez (2009). *My Anxious Mind: A teen's guide to managing anxiety and panic.* Washington, DC: Magination Press

General Parenting

Websites

fosteringresilience.com

Resources, information and books for teens and parents on building resilience. (US)

theparentingplace.com

Resources, webinars, books, events, workshops, courses and advice to help you gain insights, perspective and confidence in parenting your teen. (NZ)

Books

The following New Zealand and Australian authors have written a number of great books that are easy to read and offer helpful and humorous information, tips and techniques on raising teenagers:

Michael Carr-Gregg, Nigel Latta, Diane Levy, Celia Lashlie and Ian & Mary Grant.

Moreno, M. (2013), *Sex, Drugs 'n Facebook: A parents' toolkit for promoting healthy internet use.* Berkley: Hunter House Inc.

Other Areas of Concern

Many of the mental health and youth sites noted above will contain information about the below areas or links to appropriate websites. Other links that may be of use include:

BULLYING: onevoice.net.nz; kidspot.co.nz; cyberbullying.org.nz

EATING DISORDERS: ed.org.nz; nedc.com.au

INTERNET SAFETY: cyberbullying.org.nz; netsafe.org.nz; urge.co.nz

SEXUALITY: rainbowyouth.org.nz; outline.org.nz

SUBSTANCE ABUSE: alcohol.org.nz/alcohol-you/alcohol-your-kids; alcoholdrughelp.org.nz/youth-service

SUICIDE and SELF-HARM: spinz.org.nz; conversationsmatter.com.au; lifeline.org.nz

Phone, Text and Email Supports

Alcohol Drug Helpline: 0800 787 797

Depression Helpline: 0800 111 757

Kidsline: 0800 543 754 (near-peer telephone counselling service supporting children up to 14 years old; available 4 to 6 p.m. weekdays)

Lifeline Aotearoa: 0800 543 354

OUTline: 0800 688 5463 (confidential support for sexuality or gender identity issues)

Tautoko (suicide helpline): 0508 TAUTOKO (0508 828 865)

the lowdown: free text 5626; email team@thelowdown.co.nz (12 noon to 12 midnight)

What's Up youth helpline: 0800 WHATSUP (0800 942 8787) (1pm–11pm; free counselling for young people)

Youthline: 0800 376 633, free text 234, email talk@youthline.co.nz

Index

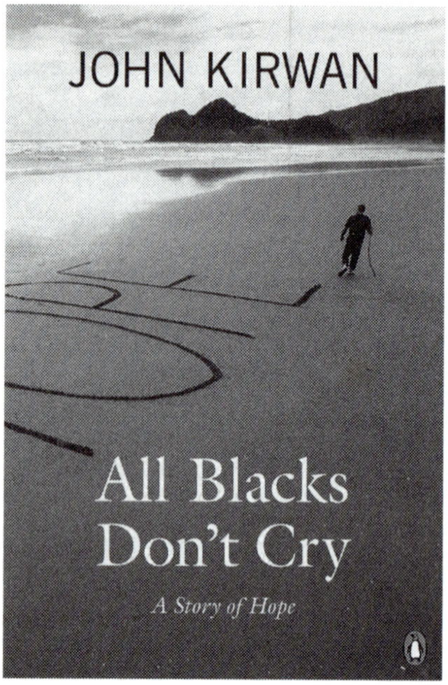

Over 40,000 copies sold

A prominent and revered figure at the dawn of the professional age of rugby, John Kirwan seemed to live a charmed life.

But nobody knew that behind closed doors he was living a life of torment. Afflicted with depression for many years – including those as a high-profile sportsman – Kirwan was able to survive by reaching out, seeking help from those closest to him.

All Blacks Don't Cry is John Kirwan's story of hope, of working through the pain and living a full life. It is a poignant, inspirational and helpful example for anybody battling depression.

'May be the most useful book ever written by a New Zealand rugby player.'
—Philip Matthews, *Weekend Press*

Also available as an ebook